CW01334004

Carol Lefevre has published nine books, as well as short fiction, essays and journalism. Her novella *Murmurations* was shortlisted for the 2021 Christina Stead Prize for Fiction in the NSW Premier's Literary Awards, and the Fiction Prize in the 2022 South Australian Festival Awards for Literature. She holds a PhD in Creative Writing from the University of Adelaide, where she is a visiting research fellow. She lives in Adelaide, where she tends a small garden of fruit trees, roses and herbs.

BLOOMER

CAROL LEFEVRE

affirm press

affirm press

First published in Australia in 2025 by Affirm Press, a Simon & Schuster (Australia) Pty Limited company
Bunurong/Boon Wurrung Country
28 Thistlethwaite Street, South Melbourne VIC 3205

Affirm Press is located on the unceded land of the Bunurong/Boon Wurrung peoples of the Kulin Nation. Affirm Press pays respect to their Elders past and present.

New York Amsterdam/Antwerp London Toronto Sydney/Melbourne New Delhi
Visit our website at www.simonandschuster.com.au

AFFIRM PRESS and design are trademarks of Affirm Press Pty Ltd, Inc., used under licence by Simon & Schuster, LLC.

13 5 7 9 10 8 6 4 2

Text copyright © Carol Lefevre 2025
Artworks copyright © Margaret Ambridge 2025

All rights reserved. No part of this publication may be reproduced, stored in a retrieval system, or transmitted in any form or by any means, electronic, mechanical, photocopying, recording or otherwise, without prior permission of the publisher.

A Cataloguing-in-Publication entry for this book is available from the National Library of Australia

A catalogue record for this book is available from the National Library of Australia

9781923293038 (hardback)
9781923293861 (ebook)

Cover design by George Saad © Affirm Press
Typeset by J&M Typesetting in Garamond Premier Pro
Printed and bound in China by RR Donnelley Asia Printing Solutions Ltd

FSC MIX Paper FSC® C144853

The paper this book is printed on is from FSC®- certified forests and other controlled sources.
FSC® promotes environmentally responsible, socially beneficial and economically viable management of the world's forests.

For Christopher

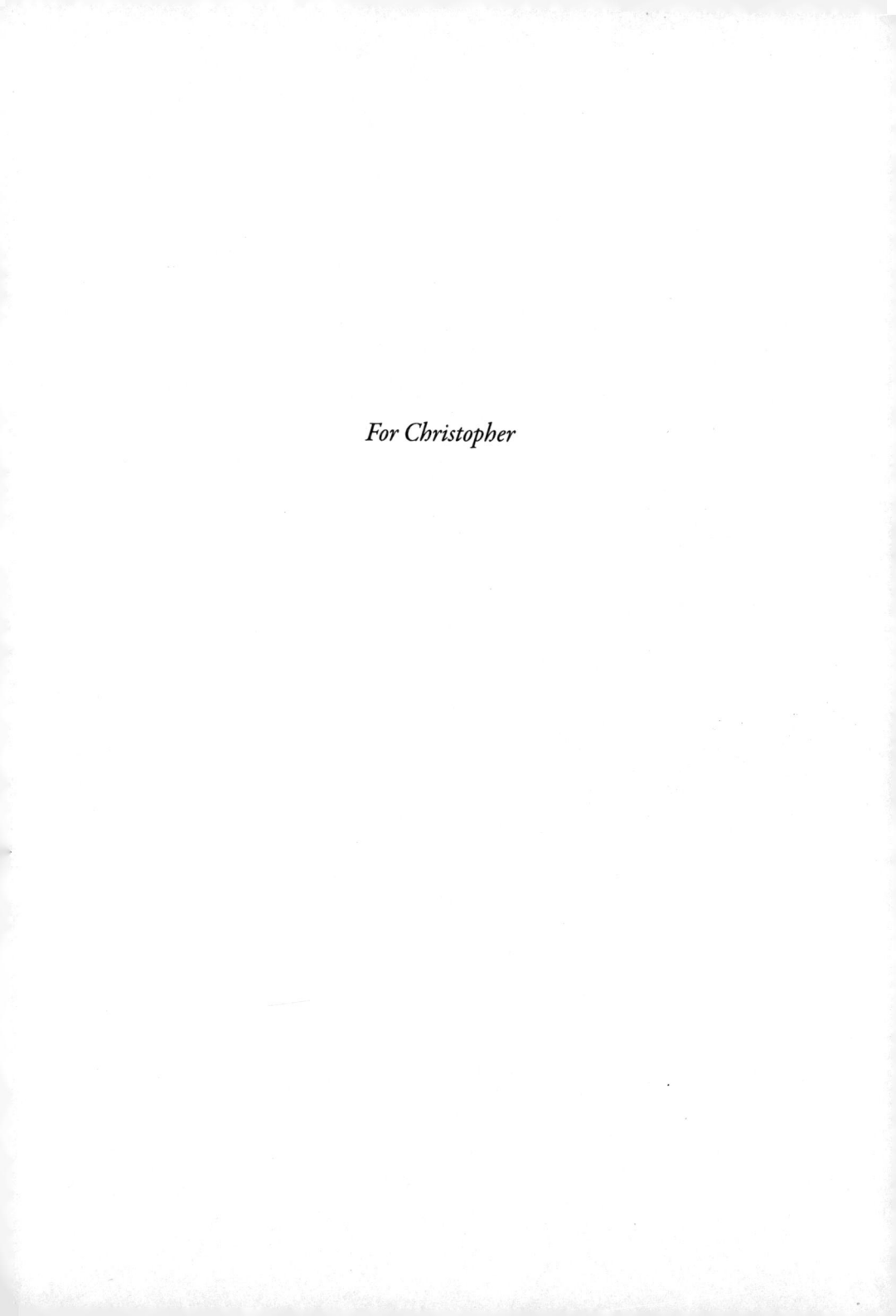

Contents

Prologue	Going Forth	1
Part I	**Summer**	**9**
Chapter 1	Full Bloom	11
Chapter 2	Gathering Flowers, Weaving Garlands	28
Chapter 3	Homesick for Ourselves	40
Chapter 4	Disappearing Acts	53
Part II	**Autumn**	**61**
Chapter 5	Death Cleaning	63
Chapter 6	Things Fall Apart	71
Chapter 7	Past and Future in Every Moment	81
Chapter 8	The Possibility of Radiance	92
Part III	**Winter**	**103**
Chapter 9	When Enough Is Enough	105
Chapter 10	Saying Goodbye	119
Chapter 11	Lost in Time	123
Chapter 12	Love and Age	137
Chapter 13	The View from the Tower	150
Chapter 14	Finding Shelter	162

Part IV	**Spring**	**173**
Chapter 15	Imagined Gardens	175
Chapter 16	Russian Dolls and Roses	185
Chapter 17	The Ordinary and Extraordinary	196
Chapter 18	The Homeward Star	206
Chapter 19	Life After Life	218
Chapter 20	Okay, Bloomer	223

Appendices	**235**
We Need to Talk About Ageing	237
List of Artworks	266
Bibliography	268
Acknowledgements	276

> My body wanes, my mind waxes:
> in my old age there is a coming into flower.
>
> Victor Hugo

Prologue

Going Forth

According to the story in the Book of Genesis, life began in a garden. It was an earthly paradise, a place of beauty and abundance, and its two inhabitants, Adam and Eve, were not troubled by time passing, or their own ageing. That is, until they tasted the fruit from the tree of knowledge, which they'd been forbidden to eat. Whether that fabled fruit was an apple or, as some scholars suspect, a quince, for their curiosity and transgression the pair were promptly expelled. After leaving the garden they became mortal, and clocks began to tick.

Whether or not one believes the ancient tale, time is still the enemy when it comes to our ageing, and a garden, however small, is still a piece of paradise worth cultivating. The word 'paradise' has its roots in the Old Iranian *pairi-daêza*, meaning a walled enclosure. And this is what I am fortunate enough to tend – a small enclosed garden within a smallish city, in which the outside world feels far away. But for me the walled garden's meaning has always drifted towards metaphor, descriptive not only of a space planted with roses and herbs and fruit trees, but of human consciousness, and even the physical self: I may be an old woman, but I am what I think, I am what I plant, I am what I cause to flourish.

Flourishing is much on my mind at present, as the old year creaks towards its close. For on the first day of the new year I will turn seventy. It's an age that once seemed so far in the future as to not be worth worrying about. Yet suddenly, here we are, hitting the biblical threescore years and ten. It is a long stretch of time to have lived, although I seem to have arrived here all too soon. In so many ways I feel no different from the person I've always been – still loving the things I love, constantly seeking to perfect my imperfect creations, whether it be rearranging the furniture, planning changes in the garden or working on a piece of writing. Yet it does feel strange to have lived for the greater part of a century, and to have changed so radically from my childhood self. Strange, too, to remember events that are now considered part of history – the first moon landing, the assassination of an American president, young men being conscripted to fight in the Vietnam War, to name but a few.

My own ageing first came under scrutiny in my late forties, a difficult and confronting time for women. Like so many before me, I experienced a sense of having suddenly become invisible, and for a while – in a state of quiet shock – I wondered how I was to manage. At the time, I was already juggling other difficulties – chronic homesickness, a fraught relationship with an adopted child – and the last thing I needed was this nebulous sense of having lost myself somewhere along the way, never mind the night sweats and the hot flushes. Stressful doesn't come close to describing the sorrow and anxiety of those years and yet somehow they were weathered.

But seventy feels different. Seventy calls for a facing up to the certainty that time is short, and it raises many questions. Such as, am I old now? Yes, I am. Should I have a sensible haircut? No, never. I'm going to lose people and things I love: how will I bear it? You'll bear it as you've always borne your losses, one day at a time. After seventy, will I go forth as an old woman? Yes, it's time. And how then shall I define myself to others? Will I be an elder, older, a senior or simply (and this is my preference) an Old Woman? Because putting 'old' and 'woman' together in a sentence in our culture usually implies an insult, and the rebel in me wants to challenge that.

Then there are the darker questions, fearful thoughts that arise when I'm sitting with a cup of tea on the veranda after a weeding session, or by the fire on a winter's afternoon, when the house is so quiet that I can hear the tireless *tick-tick* of the mantlepiece clock. Will I live, as my mother did, into extreme old age? And if I do, will I be able to care for myself? What will I do if I get dementia? When and how will I die? What happens after death, and is there a form in which the thing people call a soul – for want of a better word – lives on, unfettered by this aged body? These life-and-death matters put the angst of my forties and fifties in the shade, though at the time it was all-consuming.

Perhaps better questions to ask now would be: How shall I make the most of this time I've been gifted by not dying young? How can I stay well, and live in my own home until my time on earth is over? How can I continue to find purpose in my life in its final stages? Will the love and happiness I've experienced over my lifetime sustain me to the end, even if the end is painful?

Most daunting of all is the prospect of ageing in a time and place that does not value old people. Here and now, in Australia, the ratio of old to young in our population is slowly tipping towards old, and this looming imbalance casts old people as a burden, a problem to be solved, or even the cause of the inflation bringing tough economic times. The subliminal message is that old folk may once have had their uses, but now it's time for them to vanish into retirement villages and aged-care homes, to be seen and heard no more. The invisibility old people are made to feel is something most older women will already be familiar with, an uncomfortable reprise of an earlier experience.

While pondering the private and public consequences of ageing, my strategy has been to retreat into the garden. A garden moves to its own rhythms, so that time is more fluid and forgiving there than in the relentless press of daily life. As a forward-looking pastime, gardening counters depression, it bolsters optimism, and the cyclical nature of the seasons passing through a patch of soil – the reassuring promise of return – brings comfort.

Perhaps no other group of people is so in need of garden therapy as those of us contemplating the more than half-empty glass. Research has shown that getting our hands into the soil boosts serotonin levels, and that serotonin, a natural antidepressant, strengthens the immune system. Contact with the soil bacteria *Mycobacterium vaccae* triggers the release of serotonin in the brain, and when we harvest edible plants there is also a release of dopamine. Researchers hypothesise that this latter response has evolved over nearly 200,000 years of hunter-gathering, so that when food is found, a flush of dopamine in the brain's reward centre triggers a state of bliss, or mild euphoria.

It is worth noticing that whatever the weather, however extreme, plants and birds are never false, never anything but themselves, and we, too, can be at ease around them. For this alone, especially as we age, we can benefit from spending time outdoors. In some countries – notably New Zealand and Canada, doctors are now offering green prescriptions, periods of time to be spent in nature rather than medication. In Finland, five hours a month is considered a minimum dose to restore health and wellbeing, while Japanese clinicians have been recommending *shinrin-yoku* or 'forest bathing' since 1982. In the United Kingdom, in 2020, the government committed £4 million to a two-year green prescription pilot as part of its post-Covid recovery plan.

How much of the way we hold ourselves is an unconscious response to the critical gaze of others? I have often caught in myself this false self being shaped by a desire to please, and to be seen. But it is only as I approach my seventy-first year that I am able to acknowledge how the mirror of other people's gaze mostly reflects a distorted self-image. Here at life's last knockings, all that matters is what *I* think and feel and believe.

During the greater part of the century I've lived through, life has changed beyond anything my young self could have envisaged. It's faster; in theory people are more connected, yet in practice they're more isolated. Old people, especially, can feel overlooked and alone in this fast-paced era. Yet at seventy we are considered to be in Young Old Age rather than Old Old Age. These are the years when most of us have fewer responsibilities, adequate finances and sufficiently good health to pursue our interests. The Young Old perform well in attention, memory and crystallised intelligence, which is the accumulated knowledge we retain and our ability to apply it in the present. We are closer to people in midlife than those aged eighty-five and older, and are less likely to require long-term care, to be dependent or poor, and are more likely to be married, living independently and working for pleasure rather than income. Overall, many studies have shown that those in this life stage experience a greater sense of happiness and emotional wellbeing than in any other period of adulthood.

For too long we've been fed an ageist narrative of decline and decrepitude, of ageing as a road that only runs downhill. But those of us who belong to the generation known as Boomers were part of the cultural revolution of the 1960s and the Second Wave of Feminism. We marched against the Vietnam War; we were the first generation to be liberated by the contraceptive pill from the fear of unwanted pregnancy. As a demographic, we are not as compliant as our parents and grandparents, whose lives were constrained and shaped by two world wars and by the Depression years of the 1930s. Our young ears were pressed to transistor radios that pumped out protest songs, and even now, while we may have lost or abandoned the long hair of our youth, and our peace-and-love-driven idealism may have taken some hard knocks, plenty of us are still engaged in various forms of activism – after all here am I, at seventy, devoting precious years to raising awareness about ageism.

Ours will be the first generation to enter aged care with laptops and mobile phones; we'll have messaging and social media, so that if we are not treated well in there, people will hear about it. Nevertheless, there are few signposts along the route from midlife to Old Old Age, and as I find ways to navigate it, I know that I will never have had greater need of the beautiful ordinary, the everyday splendour and moments of quiet connection with those I love and with the natural world. So, as the year unfolds, I plan to spend as much time as possible in the garden, thinking, reading, writing, learning to accept and welcome within myself the presence of that figure from fairy tale – the Old Woman, the Hag, the Crone.

Part I
Summer

As summer neared, as the evenings lengthened, there came to the wakeful, the hopeful, walking the beach, stirring the pool, imaginations of the strangest kind – of flesh turned to atoms which drove before the wind, of stars flashing in their hearts, of cliff, sea, cloud, and sky brought purposely together to assemble outwardly the scattered parts of the vision within.

To the Lighthouse, Virginia Woolf

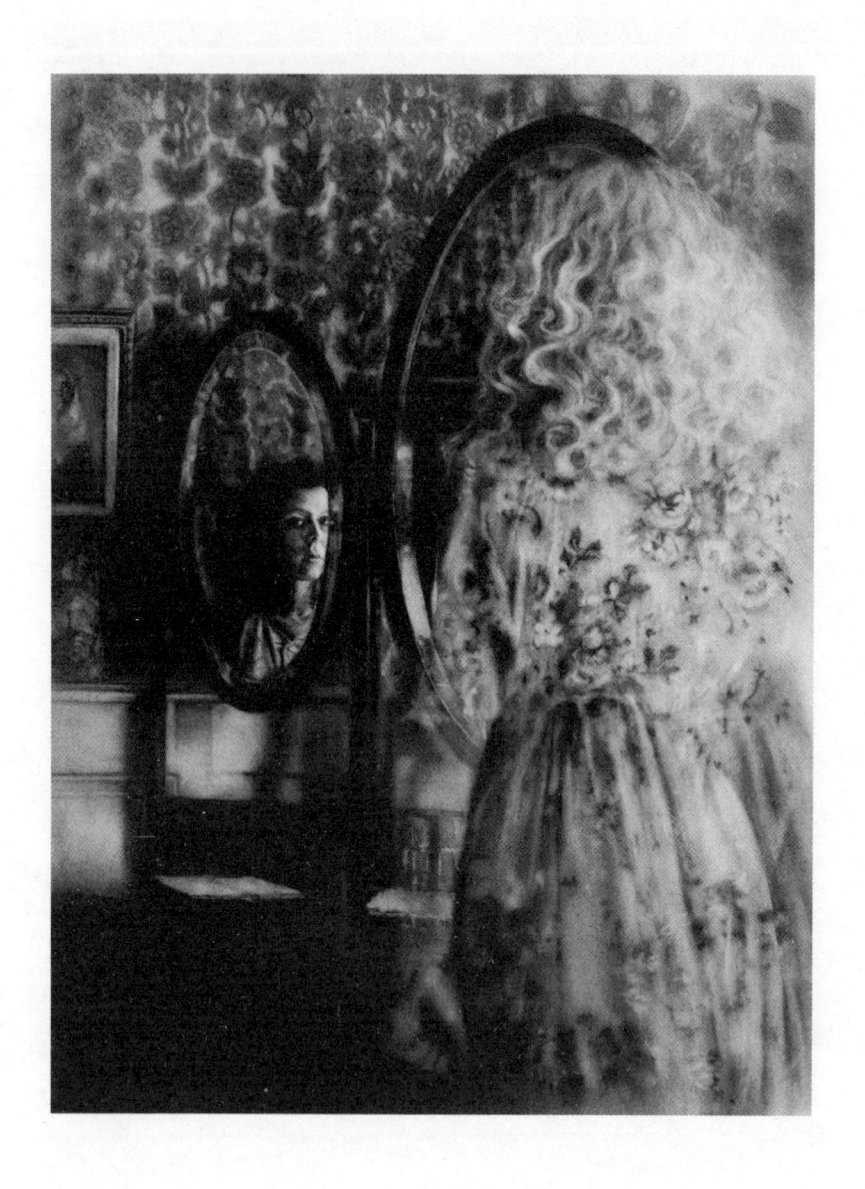

Chapter 1

Full Bloom

My birthday falls on the day of clean slates and resolutions, a day that often fulfils a forecast of brimstone-hellish heat. JD Salinger, EM Forster, Alfred Stieglitz and Maria Edgeworth are among the famous born on 1 January, but in life I rarely meet anyone who shares my birthday or anyone who would want to. As a child, this turning of my age with the turning of the year gave each New Year's Day added gravity; I might even have believed, back then, that to be born on the first day of the year was auspicious.

In my teens, and interested in astrology as so many of us were in the 1960s, I read that those born under my sign of Capricorn tend to age backwards. Astrologers agreed that Capricorns flourish as they approach old age, that they appear old when they are young and young when they are old, and my black-and-white baby photographs, with their images of an unusually wizened and serious small creature, did not contradict this theory.

As for all teenagers, my old age felt as distant as the planet Saturn that is said to rule Capricorn. Named for the Roman god of agriculture, and of time, Saturn, with its relentless twenty-nine-year orbit of the sun and its nine beautiful icy rings, is the last of the planets in our solar system that is visible to the naked eye; Saturn marks the border of all that can easily be seen from Earth, and beyond it the universe reels away into realms of darkness and uncertainty.

As the sixties gave way to the seventies my interest in astrology waned. Yet the promise of old age bringing a blossoming rather than a decline remained a comfort, which I squirrelled away as a private, self-nourishing belief. And, despite its origins in an unprovable system of planetary influence, the important thing is that, having been primed with a positive message about ageing, I feel only minimal resistance to it.

But even with my willingness to embrace each year as it comes, this next birthday feels momentous and more than a little surreal. There are moments in which I am startled to have come so far and shocked at the speed with which I've arrived here. I shake my head: how did this happen? At seventy I can no longer consider myself an 'older woman', that fuzzy descriptor within which I have so often sheltered. Perversely, this pleases me. Saturn's message is said to be that we each have to undertake a reckoning with age. But this is not really Saturn's message, it is life's message: if we live long enough, we will have to learn how to be old.

As with many of life's most important lessons, no one has prepared me for ageing; I've had to come to it alone. No one speaks of growing old, other than in passing banter. I even have a few friends who steer the subject away from their age whenever it is mentioned. And yet, all too aware of the shades of those who never travelled this far – family, friends, some taken by illness, others by accident, several by their own hand – I can't help but feel fortunate.

So, on the cusp of seventy, I stand before the mirror and ask myself whether the woman who stares back at me can really be the one in the old photographs. I'm thinking of a particular childhood snap, black and white and taken with a Kodak Brownie. In it, I sit on a box somewhere in the red dirt country beyond Broken Hill, clasping a worn cloth rabbit. It was taken so long ago that not even the faintest residue of that day remains in memory. With a lifetime between us, all that the child in the photograph and I still share are dark brown eyes and the air of seriousness with which she once looked out towards an incomprehensible future.

In *Old Age*, Simone de Beauvoir's exhaustive study of ageing, she writes that 'knowingly or not, we prepare a given old age for ourselves at the beginning of our lives: chance, and particularly biological chance, may distort it; but in so far as it depends upon the individual, he has defined his old age by his way of life'. I can only trust that my preparation has been adequate, and that chance will be kind. Seventy is a significant border, and if it can be crossed, it must be crossed. Once on the other side, I will be old, no question.

~

When I was a child, the old people around me seemed to have been old forever. As far as I knew, their hair had always been white or silver, their bodies a little too stout, their chins and arms and bellies a little too soft and saggy to be considered youthful. They were our family's last visible frontier, beyond which lay legions of ancestors I could never meet and could not envisage. I had no images of my grandparents as younger, fitter people; if I had thought about it at all I might have concluded that they were born old. Yet when I look back to those decades when my grandparents were still alive, and for periods of time I lived with them, it is sobering to realise that they were younger then than I am now.

I never heard them complain about getting older; they appeared to accept their ageing as part of life's natural order. They knew there were worse things to fear than acquiring a few more wrinkles. As young people, all of them had lost siblings – one had fallen in France in the Great War at only twenty-one, while others had succumbed to childhood illnesses or child-bearing. Theirs was an era when almost all sickness was treated at home; children were born at home. Doctors were only called if someone was dying.

In the days when I stayed in their houses, both grandfathers still went out to work – one to the mines in Broken Hill and the other to a clerk's position in the civil service in Adelaide. At some point they retired, yet I am sorry to say I remained oblivious to their milestones. As the years passed I had no sense of age settling ever deeper on them, although it must have. They were just themselves, their seniority respected within the family, and in the community.

In Broken Hill, my grandparents Roy and Angelina were the magnetic centre to which their family gravitated. After my own family had moved away – to Adelaide, to Mount Gambier and to Sydney – each summer we made a heat-numbed, long-distance road trip, with the car windows wound down, and it was always at their old house on the edge of town that we longed to arrive. For as long as I knew them it never once crossed my mind that some day I, too, would be old. Because as a child it seemed as if time stood still: all of us were simply who we were, who we would always be.

My parents did not seem old to me, yet neither were they young. They occupied a middle ground, a ledge of bedrock I could almost imagine hauling myself up to, given time. But then came puberty, with its confounding changes. The old people stayed old; my parents, of course, became annoying, while I was launched into the whirling, self-obsessed world of the teenager.

One of my grandfathers died during this period, of heart trouble he'd seemed to have suffered from forever. I am sad to record that his death passed over me like a rain shower – drenching one minute, and all but forgotten the next. It was the late sixties, and in Sydney I was singing five nights a week with a band. The old town on the edge of the desert felt remote as a distant planet, caught up as I was in the thrill of being immersed in music, of earning my own money, of behaving as if I were a grown-up.

Then when I was twenty-one, my father – whom I'd believed indestructible – was diagnosed with a brain tumour. He was forty-nine when he died. His passing dragged my attention back from my own concerns in a way nothing else could have done. The world felt suddenly more threatening, a place where people you loved could be snatched away from you. It would never again feel as carefree as the years before his death. But life went on, just as people said it would, even though it was different. I got up and went to work each day; I imagine I looked like a young woman who was coping, but inside I felt as if, overnight, my age had doubled.

At twenty-one I learned that, unlike death and taxes, old age is not a given. If we are lucky enough to reach it we will experience more of this extraordinary life than those who die young. And now that I have lived so much longer than my father managed, now that I am older than the beloved old ones of my childhood, I have begun to wonder at what point old age begins. Does it start at seventy? Is it the same for everyone? Having crossed into old age, are we the same person we've always been, but with wrinkles, or do the years add layer upon layer of complexity that turn us into someone else? Does being older really make us wiser? Does it make us happier? Above all, what is old age for?

I had been considering these questions through the writing of some essays, when I was contacted by a journalist who had read one of them online. She was writing a book about ageing, and during the Zoom interview that followed I learned that she was in her late forties, and that she and her friends were discovering, to their dismay, that they could no longer consider themselves 'hot'. But the thing they found most confronting was a sense of having become invisible.

My first thought was to point out that there would soon be worse things for her and her friends to worry about. But studying her pale face on the screen, hearing her outrage, I remembered the time, years earlier, when I, too, had been staring down my fiftieth birthday. It had been painful in ways I could never have envisaged during my teens and twenties. I recalled the night sweats and hot flushes, the realisation that I was no longer comfortable in my changing body.

At fifty I had already lost a parent, but for others it was often a time when their elders were beginning to experience the first serious health scares and setbacks. Those parental dramas sometimes coincided with guiding teenage children through the final years of schooling and the passage to young adulthood. I remembered fifty as an age when both men and women could find themselves caught in the crossfire of two different yet equally tormenting aspects of ageing. So while the anguish that can arise in the forties and fifties is not to be underestimated, I do look back now and wonder what all the fuss was about. Because at sixty, seventy, eighty and beyond, we will be tested in ways we could not have envisaged in our peri-menopausal and midlife crisis agitation. Seventy is a major milestone, and the years beyond bring challenges of a different order.

At seventy, we can no longer kid ourselves that we are only a little way past midlife: if seventy were a midpoint we'd see more people of 140, and while this is the aim of scientists tackling life-extension research, we're not there yet. Far from it. Currently, the longest documented human lifespan is that of French woman Jeanne Calment, who, when she died at 122 years and 164 days, was the world's oldest person. Reaching a hundredth birthday is still such a stretch that it has traditionally been celebrated with a letter from the reigning monarch.

Most of us have grown up with the notion that seventy is the lifespan a human might reasonably expect to attain. The origin of this lies in Psalm 90:10, which states: 'The days of our years are threescore years and ten'. It goes on to add that if we manage fourscore years, 'yet is their strength labour and sorrow; for it is soon cut off, and we fly away'. Psalm 90:12 suggests we must learn to number our days 'that we may apply our hearts unto wisdom'.

So I nodded companionably at the journalist on my computer screen, all the while wondering whether what appeared to be her signature style of coal black hair and scarlet mouth would soon become a problem for her.

'Yes,' I said. 'I remember how it was.'

She wasn't interested in the health scares that are common currency at seventy and beyond, most often endured alone and in silence. What she wanted was my opinion on how to refuse the invisibility, but all I could suggest was that she embrace it as a superpower.

~

Last winter, in preparation for this crossing into the seventies, I ceased colouring my hair. Going *with* the grey instead of against it had to do with the increasing difficulty of achieving a natural colour, as well as the expense and inconvenience of monthly visits to the hairdresser. That is what I told people. Instead, I was quietly putting in place this new life chapter, one in which the defences against ageing, held so tenaciously, were to be lowered.

During the transition from dyed brown to a new and surprising silver I sensed my social visibility decreased a little. This was not as much of a shock as the post-menopausal shift of interest, but all the same it registered with a small ping of awareness. Strangely, the decision to reveal my natural hair colour coincided with a fashion moment in which young women were bleaching their hair and dying it silver, at great expense for the ongoing maintenance. Why were they doing this? I wondered. Were they playing with their sense of invincibility? Were they testing prospective suitors? Were they under such laser-like pressure from the male gaze – perhaps intensified by pornography – that they were seeking refuge in the anonymity of age, even if only an illusion? Of course, being so obviously young meant their grey hair was unlikely to be real, so there was that. But while I achieved similar colour results at the cost only of enduring the awful growing-out period, I could tell from the reactions of strangers that I was somehow less than I had been, while the young, salon-tinted, silver-haired women, whether they wanted it or not, were more.

Deciding to go forth as an old woman naturally makes me wonder how other women have navigated this crossing. As always, I turn to books, to other women writers, to lean on their experience and wisdom. What I have discovered is the shocking scarcity of older women in fiction – indeed, there are so few books in which old women are the main characters that it is possible to make a list and plan to read them all.

The first puzzle about the scarcity of older women in novels is that older women, often avid readers, appear not to be seeking themselves in fiction but instead are reading the adventures of younger, thirty- and forty-something women. Is this because older women in novels have largely been reduced to stereotypes: the demented, the eccentric, the quarrelsome, the devoted yet sidelined grandmother, the meddling mother-in-law, the faded beauty, the disappointed spinster, the feisty older woman? How I have come to dislike that word 'feisty', with its sly undertone of aggression. Is it possible that older women readers do not recognise themselves among this sadly stunted troupe? Do books about younger women allow them to read through the filter of memory? Or are they so affected by the shame associated with ageing in our youth-obsessed culture that they shun the subject, both in life and on the page?

In her memoir *Ammonites and Leaping Fish*, Penelope Lively remarks that 'fiction is perhaps mainly responsible for the standard perception of the old', and that 'memorable and effective writing about old age is rare'. In the United Kingdom, a survey of more than a thousand women over the age of forty found that 51 per cent of those surveyed felt that older women in fiction tend to fall into clichéd roles, and 47 per cent felt there were not enough books about middle-aged or older women. Those that do appear are often insultingly portrayed as 'baffled by smart phones, computers, or the internet', and 56 per cent reported that they would like to see women their age portrayed as 'more active'. The survey, conducted by HarperCollins imprint HQ in conjunction with Gransnet, a social media platform for older people, found that women over the age of forty-five buy more fiction than any other age group.

So where in fiction, I wonder, are the good, wise, elegant women, familiar to me in real life, the capable women doing what they do with competence and compassion – managing families, and businesses, writing books and research papers, acting as mentors and role models, sustaining their even more aged parents, supporting children in their fledgling adult lives? To find a place in fiction it appears that older women must be less than they actually are; they must be cardboard characters with 'big hearts' and 'irresistible flaws'. But why should such qualities be demonstrated by older women any more than by younger women? Is it to compensate for their perceived loss of beauty, their waning sexual appeal, their post-menopausal inability to bear children? Whatever the answers, it appears that older women are some of the most underwritten and marginalised people in contemporary Western culture.

It is fair to say that men and women experience ageing differently. With their history of dominance, men have traditionally fared better than women, who suffer the fallout from both an idealisation of youth and the premium placed on feminine beauty. Bearing the burden of a view that equates beauty with youth has made women notoriously reticent about admitting their years, and almost nothing generates so much resistance and dread as when we are asked to publicly state our age, especially in a career context.

As with puppies and kittens, to be beautiful when one is young is almost guaranteed, while beauty in age may be less straightforward. The pressure on young girls that, even before puberty, results in their sexualised appearance is the same pressure that at the other end of life insists that women 'of a certain age' must resist ageing. From the battalions of expensive 'age-defying' face creams in the makeup aisles to the absence of older women in the media, the message women internalise over a lifetime is that to grow old is an admission of failure. Even the coyness of the phrase 'a certain age' delivers a coded warning, and, if we are being honest, most of us hope that with luck and decent lighting we can pass for being younger. Yet I have seen images of old women so luminous, so ripe with life, and with the powerful traces of time on their faces, that tears have sprung to my eyes in response.

I was around thirteen when, on a rare trip to Melbourne, my mother took me into one of the big department stores, where we cruised the cosmetics aisles. After the small rural town we'd travelled from it seemed the height of glamour, with its marble floors and oversized floral displays, its slender black-clad young women, all with perfect makeup. At the consultation my mother arranged at the Coty counter, where my skin type was diagnosed as 'combination', I was offered a cleanser, a toner and a moisturiser. I had exquisite skin, the consultant said, and needed to use these products morning and night. I also came away with a compact of pressed face powder, which, looking back, I hardly needed.

Memory tells me there were no products labelled 'anti-ageing' back then, whereas now they fill shelf space, not just in the makeup aisles of department stores, but in chemists and supermarkets. The term 'anti-ageing' arrived sometime in the 1980s, devised as a marketing tool to promote skincare products to older women. Its use is now ubiquitous in an industry that preys on women's insecurity, and encourages a mindset in which ageing is undesirable, a condition to be battled with expensive creams and serums.

Decades ago, Susan Sontag wrote about the double standard in ageing in which men became 'distinguished' while women became 'old bags'. Far from being superficial, or cosmetic in nature, sex-ageism can have an impact on women's ability to survive. Alarmingly, older women make up the new demographic joining the ranks of the homeless.

In 1970 Simone de Beauvoir wrote of female ageing as the 'shameful secret', and decades of feminism have wrought little change. From menopause onwards, women, like the journalist who contacted me, report becoming transparent, until eventually they realise that old women are widely regarded as diminished beings, and that our youth-driven culture harbours a deep revulsion for the age-altered female body.

To be fair, men also suffer. If Madonna has been accused of a 'lack of dignity' for performing beyond her sixtieth birthday, there are many who would silence Mick Jagger and the Rolling Stones – a band that still fills stadiums across the globe – simply because they are old. The ageing Yeats said that being old made him 'tired and furious'. French writer and politician Chateaubriand declared old age 'a shipwreck', while the poet Pierre de Ronsard, disgusted by his withered body, wrote, 'I have nothing left but bones.' Plenty of men feel driven to deny their age, and this is evident in attempts at comb-overs, in the business of hair-transplants and regrowth or the pre-emptive shaved heads of recent decades. Botox is now also marketed to men, as are anti-ageing skincare products.

To grow old in our culture, which does not value old people, is unnerving. Yet ageism is nothing new: Shakespeare wrote, 'Youth I do adore thee, age I do abhor thee.' While the old people of my childhood never complained about their own ageing, they held attitudes towards it and were quick to judge others. Phrases like 'mutton dressed as lamb' and 'over the hill' would be delivered through pursed lips; heads would shake over any woman deemed to have 'let herself go'. There might be a grudging acknowledgement that someone looked 'good for her age', but only if she was behaving in a manner deemed age-appropriate. Such criticisms were only ever aimed at women.

Growing out my hair colour has not been without anxiety, and many bad hair days. In the beginning even my mother was against it and warned me I would be sorry. To kickstart the process, my hairdresser suggested I go lighter all over to minimise the contrast between the dyed ends and grey roots. His advice was sound, but I resisted. I have never wanted blond hair; it makes me look ill. And this was the point at which anxiety kicked in, for how ill would I look, I wondered, when my hair was grey?

The whole episode reminded me of Jean Rhys's novel *Good Morning, Midnight*, in which the protagonist Sasha Jensen describes a similar 'transformation act'. Sasha's hairdresser says, 'In your place, madame, I shouldn't hesitate. But not for a moment. A nice blond cendré.' Later, Sasha mercilessly mimics the man: 'But blond cendré, madame, is the most difficult of colours. It is very, very rarely, madame, that hair can be successfully dyed blond cendré.' And which of us hasn't known such a hairdresser?

From a manual on hair-colour theory, I learn that molecules of blue pigment sit closest to the cuticle in the hair shaft, and that blue is the easiest pigment to remove. Red pigment, sitting deeper in the cortex, is more resistant. Yellow sits deepest of all, and is therefore the hardest to shift, which is why bleached hair often looks brassy, and white hair can take on a yellow cast. In both cases the yellow must be neutralised with violet.

I have resisted the yellow pigment in my greying hair. Violet shampoo keeps it at bay, but the experience has given me an insight into the much-mocked 'blue rinse' matrons of years gone by: poor souls, they were only women dealing with ageing, battling yellowing hair with fewer products than are now available.

Older women need a mature doctor and a young hairdresser: while a younger doctor is likely to judge one so ancient as to be hardly worth treating, an older doctor may have experienced some of the same aches and pains. If this sounds extreme, consider that the ageism in the general population cannot be assumed absent from those in the medical profession. As for old hairdressers, my theory is that they may be jaded after decades on their feet all day, more likely to give the same cut they have carved out many thousands of times before. Or if you should ask, God forbid, for 'something different' the result will send you home weeping, and a lot poorer. Newly minted hairdressers are trained in the latest techniques, some of which are useful in easing the transition to natural colour.

I found my new young hairdresser on Instagram, where her posts of graceful, loose updos looked like styles I might soon aspire to. For without the dye, the condition of my hair improved so radically that I resolved to grow it long. In the grey-hair movement on Instagram there are communities of women dedicated to supporting each other through their transition. Their photographs of hair in every imaginable shade and patterning of grey raise hope that social media is the perfect tool for this new women's movement, one that could be instrumental in chipping away at our damaging beliefs about ageing, and at ageism in the wider population.

While I was primed to believe I might age backwards, the example of empowered ageing set by this brave new wave of Instagrammers will surely alter the way their daughters and granddaughters deal with greying hair – indeed, many of them say that their aim is to adjust perceptions around beauty for future generations. If the movement catches on, it should give young women a confidence that was not modelled for me or my friends by the dye-dedicated, age-denying generation that preceded ours.

The gardener in me observes how some roses grow more beautiful with time. For example, the Leonardo da Vinci, an intricately pleated rose that starts out a clear strong pink and gradually evolves to a dusty colour and texture even lovelier than the fresh young blooms. Why can't we humans age in the same manner?

Aside from a handful of novelists, no one offers clues as to how one's old age might be managed. In searching for answers to my own ageing I have settled in to a pattern of thinking, reading and writing that is not unlike the patterns a spider makes in spinning a web between rose bushes – the hundreds of small, tidy, tying-in movements; the occasional bold free-fall into space. I am taking the view that ageing is a necessary adventure, and at seventy I will write what only an old woman *can* write. Not because I am unusually wise, but because I *will* be old, and I want to understand what old age is for.

A blackbird has been sitting on four beautiful turquoise eggs in the topiary bush outside my bedroom; it is her last clutch of the summer, and I have been hoping that the chicks will not hatch during the worst of the heat. But they emerge to a burning wind and dry lightning, on an end-of-the-world kind of day, with a top of forty-six degrees. Mama bird perches on the edge of the nest so as not to add her body warmth to the already knock-out temperature.

Twice a day I spray the courtyard with water, and somehow these blind scraps of life survive to open their eyes, to grow feathers, and fill the nest. For the parent birds, foraging in the heat must be exhausting, and when the male hops down from the brush fence to poke about on the lawn he looks ruffled and worn.

Within days of hatching, it seems, the baby birds are getting ready to leave the safety of the topiary bush. I watch the last of them as it sits with fluffed feathers, apprehensively contemplating the momentous leap. The parent bird makes encouraging noises from a nearby tree, but the baby seems reluctant. Then, without warning, it flutters to the ground. Who knows what it is that makes the moment right to go?

Extract from my garden journal, January 2021

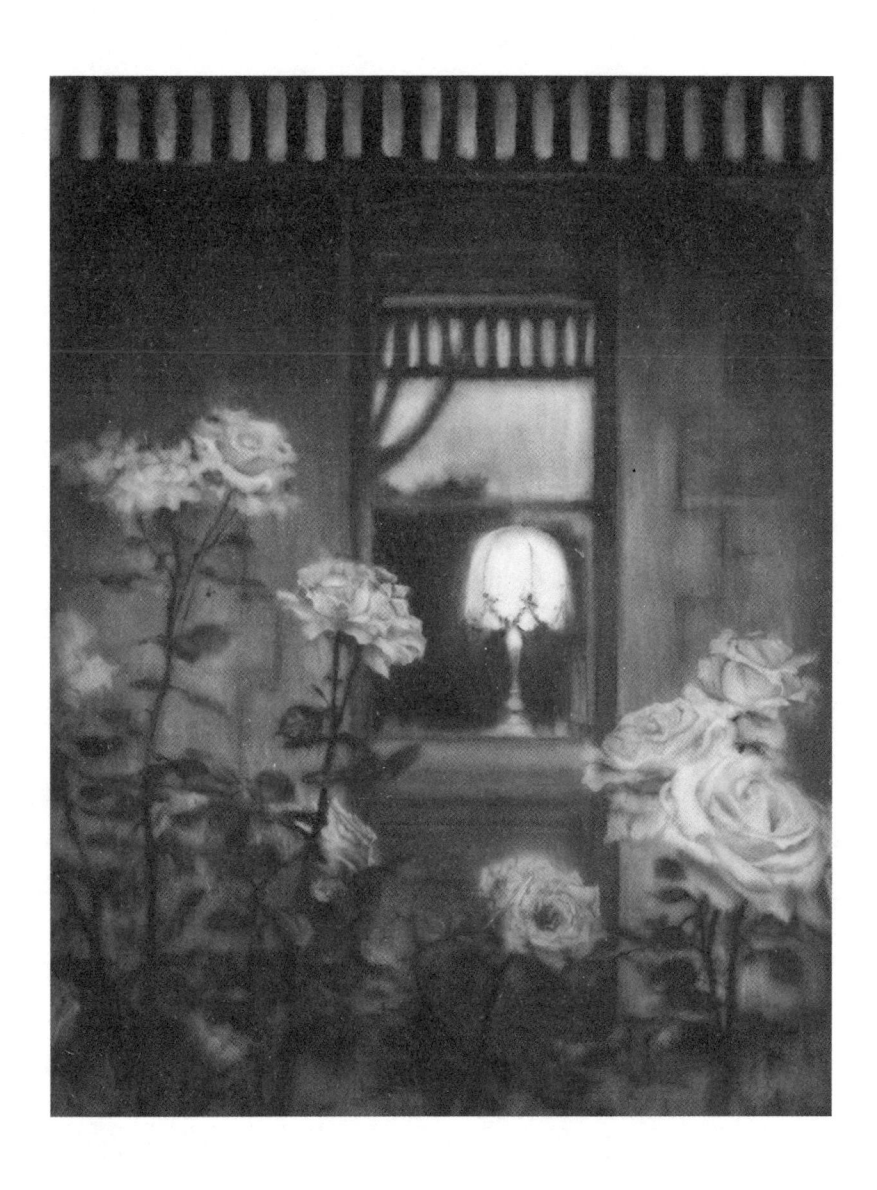

Chapter 2

Gathering Flowers, Weaving Garlands

Only sixteen days after my seventieth birthday, life has changed forever with my mother's death. At ninety-five, her loss at some point was to be expected, yet the suddenness with which death has swooped on her is shocking: one minute we were eating quiche and salad and watching the cricket, and the next we were speeding through the streets in an ambulance with lights and sirens.

Her last words to me were, 'I'd like a big glass of water to have by my bed.'

I went to the kitchen to get it for her, and then, as she was cleaning her teeth, I asked if she could manage the rest of her bedtime routine without my help. She nodded. A couple of seconds later, walking away, I heard the soft thump as she hit the floor. She would never regain consciousness, and twenty-four hours later, in the hospital, the stroke she'd suffered ended seventy years and sixteen days of her constant, loving attention.

With her passing I've lost a support that was always stronger than I knew, and which I leaned on more than I ever realised. In her quiet way she was a one-person cheer squad. A champion of my writing, she read everything I wrote at least twice, and sent out copies to her friends, even though my books were nothing like the crime novels she was addicted to reading. Without her I am less certain of who I am and what I know – questions I thought I had settled decades ago. Even my memories feel more fluid: it is strange, and disconcerting, and for the first time I do feel old.

As mother and daughter, we were often awkward. The bond between us, although unbreakable, was punctuated with tiny knots that rubbed and irritated and sometimes made sore patches. The bond between her and my brother had no such knots, or none that I could discern. She held him close always, creating, from childhood onwards, a nub of jealousy for me to worry at.

So there we were – with an uncomplicated love between mother and son, and a sometimes prickly love between mother and daughter. But still we held together, as whole and perfect as a walnut in its shell. With her death, the nut was cracked, its tiny world exploded.

My brother remarked after she died, 'Her thoughts were always turned towards us.'

And they were, until suddenly we were orphaned.

Mothers are not made 'good' at mothering simply through having borne a child. Just as there are good mothers, there are bad mothers, even evil mothers, and mothers of every competency between these extremes. If we are fortunate, mothers become the fixed star in our universe, the ground beneath our feet. But whatever sort of human a mother may be, whatever the quality of her mothering, we have never known life without her. On losing our mothers the longest thread of our lives is broken.

How strange it is to find this once steady ground now tilted. Sometimes it happens even without a death – mothers and children become estranged. But however separate they appear, they will always be joined – by the intimacy of the shared body space before birth, by their DNA, or by memory.

I don't think it is the grief speaking, but with the loss of my mother it feels as if there is no longer a buffer between me and death. While she lived, I had an unexplainable sense of being surrounded and protected from harm. I suppose this has its roots in how she held me back from the traffic when I was a small child, or caught me by the collar as I stumbled. Now with no watchful eye, no lightning-quick hand to restrain, the world feels more dangerous, even though in the last years of her life I was the one shielding her from passing cars, or catching her by the arm.

The British painter Celia Paul, in her autobiography *Self-Portrait*, describes how the world around her felt similarly changed by her mother's death. 'All that had been structured and consoling before had broken up and dissolved.' Her mother had been the subject of many of Paul's portraits; she travelled twice a week from Cambridge to London to pose for her, until she was no longer able to climb the eighty steps to the studio. After her mother died, Paul began to paint water for the first time. 'Nothing seemed permanent, so that my subject seemed to be water.' At Lee Abbey on the Devon coast, she made studies of waves, of waterfalls and pools, of a stream after a night of torrential rain. 'I thought of grief and of how it can't be contained.'

Since my own mother's death she is a constant presence in my dreams.

It's never a dramatic appearance. She is just there, a casual participant in the slippery, sliding scenes that unfold in half-remembered rooms, or in shadowy, crowded streets. Sometimes it's her house we're in, but there are secret spaces, or the rooms are arranged as they were long ago, when her own parents were still alive. She will appear from behind the faded red velvet curtain that hung in the hallway more than fifty years ago, or move slowly among a clutter of teacups in the old kitchen, with its painted cupboards and tiny built-in table. I've never been a great believer in ghosts, but I've started to wonder whether, if they do exist, dreams are the only realm in which they can approach the living without being questioned. I'm even beginning to hope a little that this might be so, because while my mother doesn't ever say much in these nocturnal visits, on waking, the memory of her presence in the night leaves me vaguely comforted. And comfort is needed, because I'm troubled by certain aspects of her death.

There was the question from doctors about her end-of-life wishes, and whether she would want their intervention. Fortunately, I was certain that she wouldn't, having been told many times that if something brought her to this point, she wished to be allowed to go. Both my brother and I had this in writing, along with a power of attorney. But we were never asked to produce evidence that these were her wishes. The decision we made for her was simply accepted.

The scans we were shown gave no hope of recovery, or no state of recovery that she would have found acceptable. But later I wondered how often such choices favoured the family rather than the one who lay stricken, and whether proof, if it existed, should have been asked for, and given.

Troubling, too, is the memory of the twenty-four hours in which, unconscious yet still breathing, our mother was given pain relief but denied fluids. I thought of her request for that glass of water at bedtime and, fearful that we were condemning her to die of thirst, I questioned the nurses. Their answers were gentle yet evasive, I thought then, and still think now. Everything they were doing, they said, was to make her going easier.

~

Many years ago, in my mother's living room, there was a table lamp with a pink satin shade. The lamp had stood for decades in that room of the old villa, in the seaside suburb where she lived from the early 1970s, following my father's death. Originally its shade was covered with thin green silk and edged with a fringe of glass beads; it was a lamp left over from another era. But it suited the bohemian style of that room, with its high ceiling and green velvet sofas, its walls crammed with prints and paintings.

It was a room that was always dim, especially during the day in summer, when the brown holland blinds were lowered against the heat. Yet it was a welcoming room, a place where people felt free to drop in, unannounced, whenever they happened to be passing, and they were always passing. My mother would rustle up cups of tea and plates of biscuits for her stream of visitors. In winter, she'd keep a fire burning.

When the green silk perished, my frugal mother re-covered the wire frame with pink satin left over from the bridesmaids' dresses she used to sew back then to supplement her widow's pension. Perhaps the glass beads were too difficult to reattach, so instead she edged the lamp with braid.

Between each of its eight scallops she sewed a hand-fashioned satin rose flanked by two satin leaves, the same decoration she often fixed to the shoulders and hems of bridesmaids' dresses.

Voluptuously adorned, the pink lamp was occasionally poked fun at, sometimes even described as hideous, though never by me. Because in the early evenings, when it was just growing dark but the curtains had not yet been drawn, I would walk up her street, or drive over to visit, and from a block away I'd see the pink lamp shining in the living-room window. Even then it brought both a rush of pleasure and a little twist of pain, because I knew a day would come when I'd approach the house and her pink lamp would no longer glow in the dusk.

At some point I must have explained what her pink lamp meant to me, because a few years ago, when I was going through a terrible time, she gave the shade to me. At home I found a spare base, and whenever things felt bleak I would turn on the lamp. The porous nature of the satin meant the whole lampshade glowed, tinting the walls and the ceiling rose. To anyone passing along the hall when the lamp was lit, the room glowed like a magic cave. Even with my eyes closed, pink light penetrated my eyelids; after only a minute or two, my racing mind would quieten.

The mismatch of modern base and vintage shade hadn't seemed important. I told myself that when things were calmer I would search for a different base. Years passed, and I did nothing about it. But recently I resolved to find something that better suited the shade's vintage. Close to where I live is an antiques shop that specialises in period lighting; it is hung with chandeliers, packed with art deco and art nouveau lamps, and that is where I headed. When we first moved to the area fifteen years ago, the shop was run by two elderly men with old-fashioned manners. People would bring damaged lights to be repaired; their friends would drop by to drink cups of tea with them and chat. The shop, though crammed with beautiful objects, was rarely crammed with customers, but they seemed to sell enough stock to stay in business. Then a few years ago one of them died, and afterwards his partner became unwell.

I arrived to find the shop being run by the surviving owner's daughter. Her father was still living at home, she said, but suffering from dementia. She was trying to keep the place open, but it was a struggle. Within five minutes I had found not only the perfect brass base for my mother's shade, but a second pink lamp. It was ridiculously lovely, ridiculously expensive, but, mindful of the day when this repository of treasures would close, I told her I would take it.

In Paris during the Second World War, in her rooms in the Palais-Royal, Colette famously wrote under a blue lantern – not that I am in any way comparing myself to Colette. Hers was a powerful lamp with an extendable arm, fitted with a blue bulb and a shade fashioned out of the blue writing paper she favoured. Her neighbours christened the lamp *le fanal bleu*, after the beam of a lighthouse, 'a light that rakes the seas'.

They'd tell her, 'Oh, Madame Colette, you can't imagine how pretty your lantern looked yesterday, shining through the fog.'

Colette shook her head over their nosiness. 'There is nothing I can hide from them, not even the moment – at cockcrow, perhaps – when the beam from my lantern casts a blueness over the brown teapot and the white milk jug.' In her last years, the blue lantern sometimes burned early and sometimes late, for by then Colette had found little difference between night and day. For her, the hours of the night and the hours of the day, the hour for reading, the hour for writing, were all equally good.

Colette's mother, Sido, wrote in a letter to her daughter: 'I can see, my dearest, that you are haunted by the old house and its garden. This naturally gives me great pleasure, but it also makes me a little sad.'

Is there one of us that is not a little haunted by a particular house, or by a certain garden at a certain hour? I believe there is a stratum of memory reserved for such places, cherished settings from the vanished past, where cups of tea were presided over by a beloved someone.

It was under the blue lantern that Colette wrote a description of her mother at the centre of the family meal table. The table was set with Chinese cups, with stemmed glasses for the wine, and in the middle stood the 'burning cake' which Sido liked to flavour with rum.

Blue light is said to relieve anxiety; pink light in greenhouses encourages the growth of plants. Our own growth from the past towards the future is one of life's most puzzling and painful mysteries. That photograph of me at eighteen, for instance, in a tie-dyed dress and a floppy hat: how does it relate to who I am now, or to the very old woman of my possible future? Are they the same person?

Perhaps under her blue lantern Colette discovered that it is the past that anchors us. With the loving renderings of her life with Sido, she seemed to have always understood that it is the Chinese cups, the little wine glasses, the myriad details of life as it was once lived, that help us hold on to a sense of who we were and who we have become.

Of all the fragments of my mother's life of which I am now the custodian, it is not the worn-thin wedding band that is most precious, not the modest engagement ring or the ancient wristwatch that still emits a steady *tick* when wound. It is the lamp with the pink satin shade, the gorgeous, hideous, satin roses – its light, which restores me to the tinkle of teaspoons on long-vanished afternoons. A beacon that beams out of a past in which I was not yet orphaned, it bridges the abyss of my mother's absence to flood my room with a magical, possibly even healing, rose-coloured light.

There, suddenly, are the special cups, the cake crumbs, the figs, the garden flowers in jugs and vases, the winter fires, the quilts in hoops piled on chairs; and we are all there, with the blinds drawn against the heat, or with doors and windows wide to catch the faint sea breeze as we talk of books, and of art and artists. There is laughter, and companionable silence, and I am reminded that love of all these things has been my true inheritance.

As Colette wrote under her blue lantern, in the middle of another century: 'It is the image in the mind that links us to our lost treasures; but it is the loss that shapes the image, gathers the flowers, weaves the garlands.'

~

In the midst of grief I am blessed with a moment of unexpected joy when my novella, *Murmurations*, is shortlisted for the Christina Stead Prize for Fiction. When an email delivers this news I am momentarily unable to speak – caught between tears and laughter. To be listed alongside writers who are household names is beyond uplifting. No matter the final outcome, this, surely, is a late-life blooming. But it hurts, too, that I cannot share the pleasure and the honour of it with my mother.

~

I've heard that before we die, if we can speak at all, it is most often our mothers we cry out for. No matter if they were the kind of mother we hid things from, a mother we argued with and vowed never to become, a mother who embarrassed us in front of friends, or who danced wildly with us on a beach at midnight, a mother who got loud after two glasses of wine, who sang but could never hold a tune, a mother who never properly explained the facts of life but was willing to scoop us up when we fell foul of them. Of all the versions of a mother that there are, our own mother is the one that is real.

Helen Garner writes of an old man who told her that, following open-heart surgery, 'he and a ward full of other men his age woke in the dark from hideous nightmares, screaming for their mothers'. It sounds like a return to childhood, when we would wail in the night until our mother left her own warm bed and came to our rescue. For me, hers was the hand that soothed, the loving shadow that hovered over us when we were ill, the voice that whispered away night terrors. When I consider the laws of symmetry at work in the cosmos, I sometimes wonder whether, when we die, we might be returned to our mothers.

They may not be with us, yet they are within us, still. Garner writes: 'Her ghost is in my body ... My movements are hers when, on a summer morning, I close up the house against the coming scorcher, or in the evening whisk the dry clothes off the line in weightless armfuls that conceal my face.' And yes, when I roll out scraps of pastry and cut leaves and flowers to decorate a pie, when I stand in the heat-soaked garden, holding the hose, and aim a stream of water at the base of a rose bush, mother-memory moves through me like muscle-memory.

In the meantime, we must learn to live without our mothers. But without them who shall remember us as small children? Without our mothers, demons dance unchallenged in the dark. Without our mothers, we are the old ones. Speaking for myself, when night presses at the windows, I am thankful to glimpse even her ghost.

Grief works its way into my sleep. After hours of restlessness, I wake fully at four in the morning to absolute silence and a sense of loss so deep that before I know it, I am weeping. In a few hours I will rise and dress and face the strain of hosting a memorial gathering for my mother. The room is still dark when I hear the blackbird's first exploratory song. The garden, too, is dark, and I imagine him there, having left the warm cup of his nest, invisible but for the gleam of an eye, while the cold clear notes well up from his throat. His presence is a comfort, and I roll into the bedclothes, close my eyes, and am lifted for a few minutes on the melodic wave of his song.

Extract from my garden journal, February 2021

Chapter 3

Homesick for Ourselves

The hidden grief of ageing

Anyone parenting young children will be familiar with the phrase 'there'll be tears before bedtime' although its use need not be limited to the behaviour of overtired, overwrought youngsters. In a quieter, more private way, it is an expression that seems perfectly pitched to describe the largely hidden grief of ageing. Not the sharp grief that follows a bereavement, but a more elusive emotion that is, perhaps, closest to the bone-gnawing sorrow of homesickness. In *Ongoingness: The End of a Diary*, American writer Sarah Manguso evokes this sense of having travelled further from our younger selves than we could ever have imagined: 'Sometimes I feel a twinge, a memory of youthful promise, and wonder how I got here, of all the places I could have got to.'

Historically, the phenomenon of homesickness was identified in 1688 by the Swiss medical student Johannes Hofer, who named it nostalgia from the Greek *nostos*, meaning 'homecoming', and *algos*, meaning 'an ache, pain, grief and distress'. It was the disease of soldiers, sailors, convicts and slaves, and was particularly associated with soldiers of the Swiss army who served as mercenaries and among whom it was said that a well-known milking song could bring on a fatal longing, so that singing or playing that song was made punishable by death. Bagpipes stirred the same debilitating nostalgia in Scottish soldiers.

Deaths from homesickness were recorded, and for the sufferers the only effective treatment was to send them back to wherever they belonged.

The nostalgia associated with old age, if it occurs, appears incurable, since there can be no possibility of a return to an irrecoverable youth. But, as with homesickness, how badly we suffer seems to depend on how we manage our relationship with the past.

In a newsletter, the American writer Cheryl Strayed describes the process of transcribing her old journals, that, on reading one of them from cover to cover, she was left feeling:

> kind of sick for the rest of the day, as if I'd been visited by a phantom who both buoyed and scared the bejesus out of me. And the weirdest of all is that phantom was me! Did I even know her anymore? Where did the woman who'd written those words go? How did she become me?

I've experienced a similar rush of bafflement and grief upon opening a letter I'd written sometime before I turned fifty, which my mother had saved and returned to me twenty years later. Within its pages I found a younger, more energetic and vibrant self, and the realisation that this woman who inhabited the letter so vividly was no longer available to me came with a jolt of emotion that felt like a bereavement.

I was so knocked off kilter that the letter, along with others I had been planning to transcribe, had to be set aside for a day when I could muster the necessary courage and detachment. Whether that day ever comes will depend, I suppose, on how I navigate my own relationship with time, and on reaching a calm acceptance of the distance travelled.

Disbelief at the distance between the young self and the old self is one of the factors in this late-life grieving. At its root, perhaps, is an internalised ageism, innate or else massaged into us by the culture we spring from.

In a series of recent conversations with people over seventy, I encouraged them to tell their stories and to reflect on the effect of time on their lives. Childhood sometimes emerged as a place they were pleased to have left behind – and, occasionally, as a place to be held close.

Trevor emigrated alone to Australia when he was just eighteen. I asked him how often now, at seventy-five, he thinks about his childhood. 'Do you have a sense of who you were back then, and is that person still part of who you are?'

'I think about my childhood quite a lot, especially putting some distance between where I was then and where I am now,' he said. 'I didn't have a really happy upbringing, and coming to Australia was a way of getting away from home and experiencing a new culture.'

In response to the same question, Jo, at eighty-four, led me to a framed photograph, enlarged to poster-size, which has hung on the wall of both his homes. It shows him aged three, in a garden – a radiant child wearing a plain white shirt and dark shorts, arms outflung as if to embrace the natural world. He bursts with exuberance, curiosity and joy.

'I relate to that as an idea, as a concept of my life. I want to maintain that freshness, that childlike freshness. You've got no responsibilities; every day is a new day. You're looking at things in a different light, you're aware of everything around you. That's what I wanted to maintain, that feeling through my life – I'm talking age-wise. My concept of my ageing is there in that photograph.'

While older voices are often absent in the media, and in fiction they are too often presented as stereotypes, in conversation what arises can both surprise and inspire.

Penelope Lively's story 'Metamorphosis, or the Elephant's Foot', written when Lively was in her mid-eighties, explores this evolution from youth to old age through the character of Harriet Mayfield. As a nine-year-old, Harriet is reprimanded by her mother for not behaving well on a visit to her great-grandmother.

'"She's old," says Harriet. "I don't like old."'

When her mother points out that one day Harriet, too, will be old, like her great-grandmother, Harriet laughs.

'"No, I won't. You're just being silly," says Harriet, 'how can I be old? I'm me."'

If distance travelled is a factor in late-life grief, so too is a sense of paths not taken, of a younger self, or selves, that never found expression. These embryonic lives held in memory beneath the lived life are reminiscent of the pentimenti found in some old paintings – an earlier image of something that the artist decided to paint over. Art historians, using x-rays and infrared reflectography, have identified pentimenti in many famous paintings, from the adjusted placement of a controversial off-the-shoulder strap in John Singer Sargent's *Portrait of Madame X* to the painted-over figure of a woman nursing a child in Picasso's *The Old Guitarist*, and a man with a bow tie concealed beneath the brushwork of his work *The Blue Room*.

Picasso's hidden figures are assumed to be the outcome of a shortage of canvas during his Blue Period but, shortages aside, the word 'pentimento', which derives from the Italian verb *pentirsi*, meaning 'to repent', brings to these lost figures a sense of regret that resonates with the feeling in old age of having lost the younger self, or of carrying traces, deeply buried, of other lives that one might have lived.

Perhaps, too, there comes a time when the past becomes harder and harder to evoke, since there is no one living to remember it with. I felt this in my mother, that it was difficult to get her to talk about the past once she'd outlived the last of her friends and immediate family.

Sometimes she gave the strong impression that the past was a time that hadn't really existed, and, if it had, she was done with it. Yet in my recent conversations with older people, every one of them has admitted to feeling a vivid sense of the past, and of the continuing presence of a younger self. As one of them wistfully remarked, 'Sometimes she even seeps through.'

Perhaps part of the problem is the mass of ordinary detail that disappears from memory on any given day. Life is made up of so many small moments that it is impossible to hold on to them all, and if we did it might even be damaging. Imagine someone casually asking how your day had been, and responding with the tsunami of detail that those hours actually contained. After opening your eyes at first light, you'd describe your shower, your breakfast and how you slipped your keys into your handbag as you left the house; in the street you'd passed two women with a pram, a child with a small white dog on a lead and an elderly man with a walking stick. And so on.

If our minds swarmed with the trivia of daily life, more important events might be forgotten, and the neural overload might even make us ill. Yet with the realisation of the loss of these minutes and hours arises the anxiety that in time the things we do want to remember will slither away from us into the dark. I imagine this fear is one of the drivers that compels people to fill social media with photographs of their breakfasts, and of their relentless selfie-taking. It is surely the impulse behind keeping a journal.

The anxiety of losing even the passing moments in a day afflicts the author of *Ongoingness*. In it, Manguso describes her compulsive need to document and hold on to her life. 'I didn't want to lose anything. That was my main problem.' After twenty-five years of paying attention to the smallest moments, Manguso's diary is eight-hundred-thousand words long. 'The diary was my defense against waking up at the end of my life and realizing I'd missed it.' But despite her continuous effort, 'I knew I couldn't replicate my whole life in language. I knew that most of it would follow my body into oblivion.'

Is it possible that women experience grief around ageing earlier, and more emphatically, than men, given that by the age of fifty even the bodies of women who remain fit send the implacable signal that things have changed? In Alice Munro's story 'Bardon Bus', from her collection *The Moons of Jupiter*, the female narrator endures dinner in the company of a rather malicious man, Dennis, who explains that women are 'forced to live in the world of loss and death! Oh, I know, there's face-lifting, but how does that really help? The uterus dries up. The vagina dries up.'

Dennis compares the opportunities open to men with those available to women: 'Specifically, with ageing. Look at you. Think of the way your life would be, if you were a man. The choices you would have. I mean sexual choices. You could start all over. Men do.' When the narrator responds cheerfully that she might resist starting over, even if it were possible, Dennis is quick to retort: 'That's it, that's just it, though, you don't get the opportunity! You're a woman and life only goes in one direction for a woman.'

In another story in the same collection, 'Labor Day Dinner', Roberta is in the bedroom, dressing for an evening out, when her lover George comes in and cruelly remarks, 'Your armpits are flabby.' Roberta says she will wear something with sleeves, but in her head she hears the 'harsh satisfaction in his voice. The satisfaction of airing disgust. He is disgusted by her ageing body. That could have been foreseen.'

Roberta thinks bitterly that she has always sought to remedy the smallest sign of deterioration:

> Flabby armpits – how can you exercise the armpits? What is to be done? Now the payment is due, and what for? For vanity. Hardly even for that. Just for having those pleasing surfaces once, and letting them speak for you; just for allowing an arrangement of hair and shoulders and breasts to have its effect. You don't stop in time, don't know what to do instead; you lay yourself open to humiliation. So thinks Roberta, with self-pity … She must get away, live alone, wear sleeves.

Many emotions that arise around our ageing can be traced back to a fraught relationship with time. French philosopher and Nobel Prize winner Henri Bergson says, 'Sorrow begins by being nothing more than a facing towards the past.' For Roberta, as for many of us, it was a past in which we relied on those 'pleasing surfaces', perhaps even took them for granted, until they no longer produced the desired effect.

Middle age is sometimes referred to as the Age of Grief. It's when we first glimpse our own mortality; we feel youth slipping away into the past, and the young people in our lives begin to assert their independence. We have our midlife crises then; we join gyms and take up running; we speak for the first time of 'bucket lists', the term itself an attempt to diminish the sting of time's depredations. None of this will save us from the real Age of Grief, which comes later and hits harder, because it is largely hidden, and we'll be expected to get on with it in silence.

In my conversations with old people, grief has surfaced from causes other than what might be called 'cosmetic' changes. Following a severe stroke, eighty-year-old Philippa describes the pain of having to make the decision to relinquish her home and move into residential care.

'It's when you lose your garden, which you've loved, and you've got to walk away from that. I've got photos of the house, and I look at them and think, oh, I just love the way I did that room, decorated it, things like that. But change happens.'

'Somehow change always comes with loss,' I say, 'as well as bringing something new.'

'Yes. I just had to say to myself: you can't worry about it, and you can't change it. That sounds hard, but it's my way of dealing with it.'

Tucked away in residential care homes, and largely invisible to those of us lucky enough to still inhabit the outside world, elderly people like Philippa are quietly raising resilience to an art form.

In her poem 'One Art' the American poet Elizabeth Bishop advises losing something every day, from the simple annoyance of misplaced door keys to the regrettable losses of cities and countries.

While the losses elderly people commonly accumulate may be less grand, they are no less devastating. One by one they will relinquish driver's licences; for many there will be the loss of the family home and their belongings, apart from whatever will fit into a care home's single room. Perhaps they have already given up the freedom of walking without the aid of a stick or walker. There may be dietary restrictions imposed by conditions such as diabetes, or the invisible disabilities of diminished hearing and eyesight.

A failing memory, one would think, must be the final straw. And yet, what seems to be the actual final straw is a situation of feeling 'unseen' or 'looked through', where for indefensible reasons the old person finds themself being 'missed' in favour of someone younger. It might, for example, be a moment when they are ignored as they patiently wait their turn at a shop counter.

In my conversation with Philippa, she remarked that old people are often looked through when they are part of a group, or when they are waiting to be served. 'I have seen it happen to other older people, as if they don't exist. I have called out assistants who have done that to other people.'

Surely the least we can do, as fortunate beings of fewer years, is to acknowledge the old people among us. To make them feel seen, and of equal value.

'Ageism, Healthy Life Expectancy and Population Ageing: How Are They Related?' is a recent survey conducted with more than 83,000 participants from fifty-seven countries. It found that ageism negatively impacts the health of older adults; in the United States people with a negative attitude towards ageing live 7.5 fewer years than their more positive counterparts.

In Australia, the National Ageing Research Institute has developed an age-positive language guide as part of its strategy to combat ageism. Examples of poor descriptive language include terms such as 'old person', 'the elderly' and even 'seniors'. That last term appears on a card Australians receive shortly after turning sixty, which enables them to receive various discounts and concessions. Instead, we are encouraged to use 'older person' or 'older people'. But this is just another form of age-masking that fools no one. It would be better to throw the institute's energy into destigmatising the word 'old'. What, after all, is wrong with being old, and saying so?

To begin the process of reclaiming this word from the pejorative territory it currently occupies, old people need to start claiming their years with pride. If other marginalised social groups can do it, why can't old people? Some activists working against ageism are beginning to mention Age Pride.

If we become homesick for who we once were as we age, we might remind ourselves of the meaning of *nostos* and consider old age as a kind of homecoming. Because the body we travel in is a vehicle for all the iterations of the self, and the position we currently inhabit is part of an ongoing creative process. This is the evolving story of the self, which, from the 1980s, psychologists, philosophers and social theorists have been calling narrative identity.

The process of piecing together a narrative identity begins in late-adolescence and evolves across the entire life course. Like opening a Russian doll from whose hollow shell other dolls emerge, at our centre is a solid core composed of traits and values as well as the narrative identity we have put together from all the days – including those we cannot now remember – and from all the selves we have ever been. Perhaps even from the selves we might have been, but chose instead to paint over.

In 'Metamorphosis, or the Elephant's Foot' Harriet Mayfield tells her husband, 'At this point in life. We are who we are – the outcome of various other incarnations.'

We know our lives, and the lives of others, through fragments. Fragments are all we have. They're all we'll ever have. We live in moments, not always in chronological order. But narrative identity helps us make meaning of life, and the vantage point of old age offers the longest view. The story of the self carries us from the deep past to the present moment, and the great life-challenge old age appears to have set us is to maintain balance in the present while managing the remembered past – with all its joys and griefs – and the joys and griefs of the imagined future.

I am interested in the garden as a source of solace and wonder if it is only because I am old now that this works for me. Would I have felt calmed by a garden in my young days, in the midst of the dramas and sorrows that dogged me? I doubt it. I was too self-absorbed then to sit and wonder about a bird, or take comfort from seeing it come to drink at the water bowl. Would baby quinces have soothed me in the days of romantic entanglement? It's unlikely. So perhaps a garden belongs to this age of womanhood when the self becomes slightly invisible even to the self.

Extract from my garden journal, February 2021

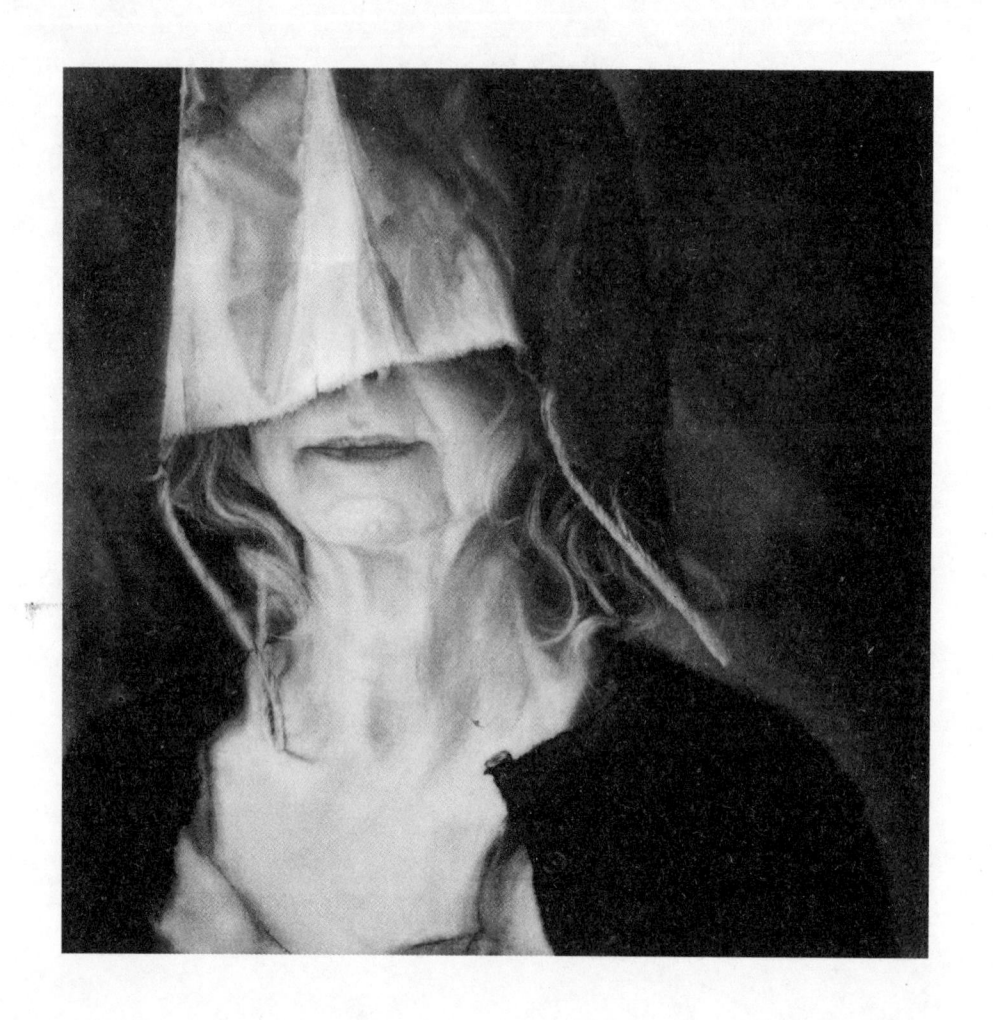

Chapter 4

Disappearing Acts

Age creeps up on us with enormous stealth; the first time I became aware of my decreased visibility it fizzed through me like a low-voltage electric shock. It was as if I had accidentally stepped behind a gauze screen – I was still visible, but eye contact was cursory, engagement diminished. After that, invisibility accelerated. I was in my late forties.

Perhaps it was the effect of menopause, the hormonal changes reflected in hair and skin and even scent. I think now of Germaine Greer's observation of the unknowable effect on women's lives of being, for so many years, under constant male scrutiny. And yes, it becomes the thing one leans on, braces against, shrinks from or yearns for, so that when it is withdrawn there must be a rebalancing. It is as if a gale-force wind has ceased to blow after years at sea: one must develop new land legs.

Young women cannot envisage this. I know I couldn't. It just never occurred to me that life would ever change. It is only with hindsight that I understand that young women are visible and old women are not. Unfortunately, this doesn't mean that the world grows safer for women as we age. Misogyny, where it exists, just leaps out at us from different hiding places; it hurls insults using another vocabulary.

In *How to Disappear*, Akiko Busch points out that if a woman is complicit in viewing herself as an *object* of the male gaze, the withdrawal of that gaze is likely to be more acutely felt. On the other hand, a *subject* experiences her own agency. She is, Busch says, 'the author of her own life'. It would seem that throwing one's effort into resisting time's changes are as misguided and as bound to fail as a seed that tries to germinate in the wrong season. Astonishingly, 'mother' plants imprint information in the genes of their seeds: memories of weather, cues about when to lie dormant and when to begin their journey towards the light. If we are to fully author our own lives, we may need to embrace the 'weather' of our ageing. We can choose to treat it as a process through which we might deepen our own inward gaze, and to intensify our observation of the outside world.

It also strikes me that invisibility might be a boon if we could only find ways to use it. I am filled with delight to learn of an artist in Victoria who uses her invisibility to engage in guerrilla acts of activism. Dr Deborah Wood began a decade ago with street art paste-ups in a lane in Ballarat. Nervous about being challenged, Wood took the precaution of wearing a hi-vis vest and had a friend spotting for her. But people walking past appeared not to see her, and Wood concluded she might even rob a bank and get away with the loot. Her drawings disrupt stereotypes about women and age, and all these years later her old women dancing in tutus, or with their mouths stretched wide in a silent scream, adorn the walls of Melbourne's Hosier Lane, among other places.

Dr Wood says, 'Perhaps by wryly donning the invisibility cloak on our own terms we can be disrupters and activists who change expectations around ageing.'

If the idea of old women dancing seems unlikely, it shouldn't, as I discovered during a conversation with ninety-year-old Jean. Jean had learned to tap-dance in childhood, and has only recently hung up her tap shoes. Before that she often took part in group performances, dancing and playing the ukelele.

The freedom to move about the world unbowed by others' expectations, and perhaps even to subtly challenge them, should not be underestimated. Germaine Greer writes:

> Only when a woman ceases the fretful struggle to be beautiful can she turn her gaze outward, find the beautiful and feed upon it. She can at last transcend the body that was what other people principally valued her for, and be set free both from their expectations, and her own capitulation to them.

She goes on to acknowledge that 'it is quite impossible to explain to younger women that this new invisibility, like calm and indifference, is a desirable condition'.

In agreeing with Greer, I am not suggesting that when the struggle for beauty ceases, the ageing woman is no longer beautiful. Beauty in age does not rely on appealing features or a flawless complexion but emanates from a capacity for patience and kindness, a depth of experience that has settled into the face and body over a long lifetime. It is evident in eyes that have witnessed history being made, witnessed history repeat itself, eyes that have mourned many losses yet remain curious. Beauty continues. What ceases is the struggle.

Even so, the removal of the gaze is what prompts most of us to become aware of our own ageing. The loss matters more to some of us than to others and, despite the freedom from surveillance that it heralds, it is still a sobering moment, a rite of passage unimaginable in youth.

Beyond sixty, women fade not only from fiction and the male gaze, but from every gaze. Younger people of both sexes do not see them; children do not see them; walking suburban streets for the good of their health, older women can find themselves budged off the pavement into the traffic. I walk every day, and each time I am bumped or forced to step aside, I long to stop the culprit and quote from Sally Vickers's novel *Miss Garnet's Angel*: 'if you are young now you might hold it in your mind that one day you too will be old'.

More ominously, older women may be less visible to their doctors, and other health professionals, and it is alarming to think that the ageing female body may not attract even their concentrated interest or concern. I remember my dismay when ABC News reported that a seventy-eight-year-old woman with a broken foot, split lip, cut nose and sprained wrist had been denied treatment at a private hospital in Hobart, despite being in possession of paid-up private health insurance. Over sixty-five, she was deemed 'too old', and her injuries too complex, to be financially viable for the hospital to treat. Fortunately, the woman had a daughter-in-law to advocate for her, and she received treatment at a public hospital, though not before she had been humiliated and made to feel unworthy of care. Many elderly men and women must face such situations alone, with a courage that is humbling.

Even more troubling is the prospect of a future in which our elderly population increases. The Australian Bureau of Statistics predicts that by 2053, 21 per cent of the population will be aged sixty-five and over (around 8.3 million people) and 4.2 per cent will be eighty-five and over (1.6 million). Inevitably, this raises concerns that the elderly will put unsustainable pressure on public funds, particularly in rising health costs. Socially, these predictions generate an angry background buzz; they pit young against old, positioning the elderly as a threat, fuelling resentment that surfaces as 'boomer bashing'.

Under international law, the elderly have a right to the 'highest achievable level of health'. However, it is not paranoid to believe that a time will come when behind closed doors in the public health system there are discussions about rationing the use of expensive medical technologies for elderly patients, and about who should and should not receive treatment and care. Perhaps these conversations have already been held.

During the early days of the pandemic, comments below news articles expressed the view that Covid-19 would likely only be fatal for the elderly, as if this were of little or no consequence. As the chaos unfolded in China, and then Italy, a letter from a group of Italian doctors reported that older patients were not being resuscitated, that they died alone without appropriate palliative care.

In the United States, critical care protocols advocated saving the maximum number of life years rather than the maximum number of lives, and their guidelines make chilling reading. In Australia, during that blighted April, as hospitals scrambled to formulate protocols the ABC reported that they would be left to make their own decisions, which meant that patients would receive different treatment at different hospitals.

Ethical considerations put forward by the Macquarie University Research Centre for Agency, Values and Ethics ruled out bias on the grounds of age, disability, having or not having dependents, social standing or perceived worth, and socioeconomic status. However, scarce resources were to be allocated based on the patient's capacity to benefit, their time to benefit and their prognosis. The decision-making flowchart for critical care admissions, if resources were under strain, made it clear that patients who would require longer intensive care treatment were to be shuffled onto a ward to die.

~

The radiance of youth cannot last; it can only be transformed into a more mature radiance. Being invisible, one may as well work at making something beautiful and, for some of us, perhaps for the first time in our lives, a garden becomes important. In myriad ways, a garden shows its gratitude to the gardener; a garden – even if it consists of a collection of potted plants – may, in the end, show more gratitude than one's children.

Sitting in the sun in her south-facing Hampstead garden, with its ripening peaches, Lady Slane, the gentle yet steely heroine of Vita Sackville-West's *All Passion Spent*, indulges in the luxury of surveying her past as 'a tract of country traversed'. Her life, she realises, has 'become a landscape', and at last she can see the whole view, can wander through it as she chooses. The garden is a place of reflection for Lady Slane, as it is for me, and for countless others. And that view of the entire landscape of one's life is the true gift of having lived a long time.

As I write this, at a cafe table, I notice the conversations in progress at other tables, in both verbal and body languages, and it occurs to me how false we often are with each other. And not only with each other but with ourselves. Strangely, I had been blind to this self-falseness – as in adopting a 'telephone voice', or behaving differently with different people – until I grew the dye out of my hair. Then, as a shining silver replaced the chemical-deadened brown, it felt like some deep truth had been revealed after years of cover-up. It was not just a physical revelation: I have found myself writing more openly; I feel more authentic in my own skin.

On visibility, I love the argument put forward by the great Victorian art critic and thinker John Ruskin as he addresses the philosophical question of the word 'blue': whether it means the sensation of colour the human eye receives upon gazing at the open sky or at a bell gentian. If the 'sensation can only be felt when the eye is turned to the object, and as, therefore, no such sensation is produced by the object when nobody looks at it, therefore the thing, when it is not looked at, is not blue'.

The same argument can be applied to other experiences, for example to whether sweetness truly exists if there is no tongue with the capacity of taste. The logical conclusion of this view is that it does not matter what things are, that their truth depends upon their appearance to, or effect upon, the viewer. 'A philosopher may easily go so far as to believe, and say, that everything in the world depends upon his seeing or thinking of it, and that nothing, therefore, exists, but what he sees or thinks of,' writes Ruskin.

I can understand how women become complicit in this view, which is an extension of the power of the male gaze. Perhaps this is one of the immeasurable and damaging effects on women's lives that Germaine

Greer referred to, after decades of being exposed to close male scrutiny. Ruskin, though, is clear:

> The word 'Blue' does *not* mean the *sensation* caused by a gentian on the human eye; but it means the *power* of producing that sensation: and this power is always there, in the thing, whether we are there to experience it or not, and would remain there though there were not left a man on the face of the earth.

He likens the power of blue to the power of gunpowder to explode.

As older women, we must apply Ruskin's reasoning to our own visibility: whether or not we are seen, we have the power of womanhood. And if when you look at us you do not see us, it is not our fault, but yours.

Part II
Autumn

And all the lives we ever lived
And all the lives to be,
Are full of trees and changing leaves
>*To the Lighthouse*, Virginia Woolf

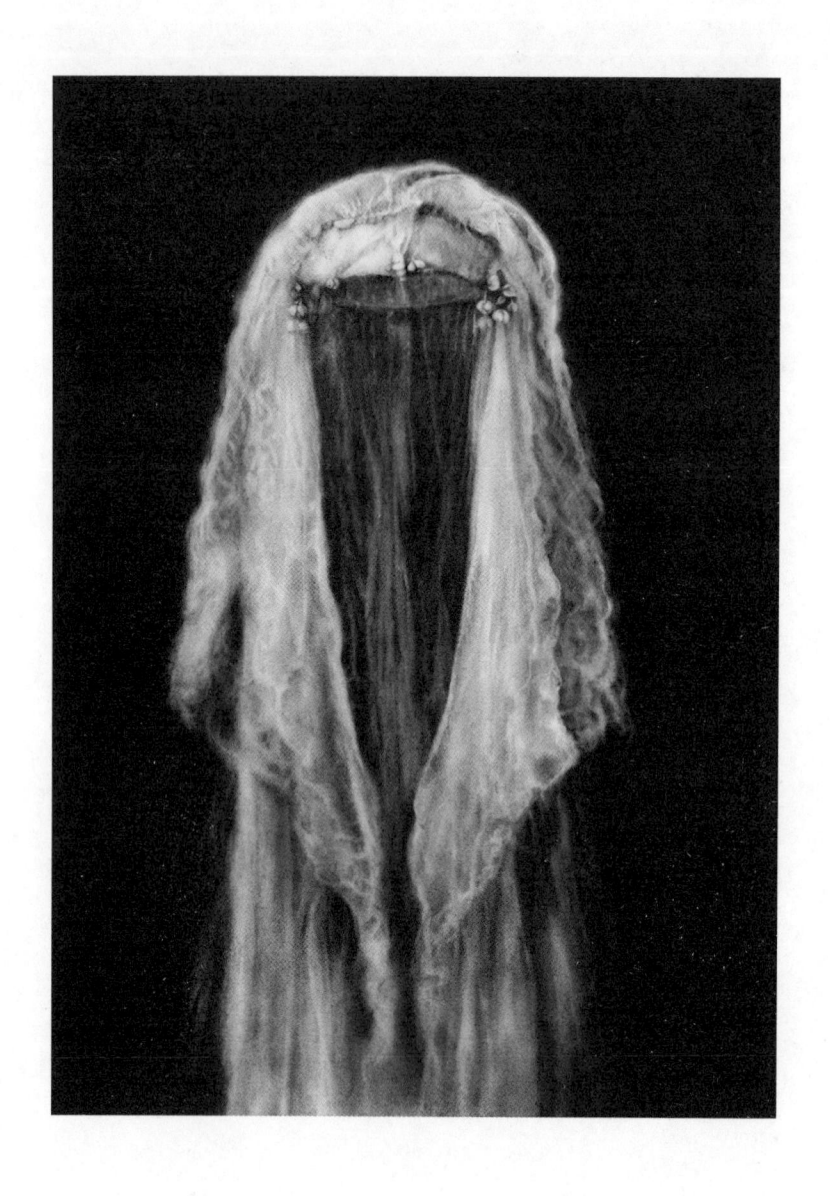

Chapter 5

Death Cleaning

In an online workshop with the American writer and teacher Natalie Goldberg, we are asked to make a list of thirty objects within our immediate line of sight. This is how my list begins: boxes of my notebooks; a green plaid chair; a portrait of me, painted by my mother; the sofa where I rest most afternoons; an old leather suitcase; a cyanotype print I made of the garden; two black-and-white photographs of my parents in silver frames; a lidded pot containing R's baby teeth; my mother's sewing machine ... the list goes on. I could write an essay on every one of these objects, its history, and how it came to be in my writing room. And while it is comforting to be surrounded by these familiar things, and all the other objects I haven't named, what is to be done with them? Are they to linger on until they become someone else's problem, or should I get started on disposing of them myself?

There has been no immediate pressure to disperse my mother's belongings. My brother and his wife are to move in to her house, but for now it is not their primary residence, so they have decided there is no need to rush. Nevertheless, I rouse myself to deal with her personal effects. My mother had done a bit of tidying herself in her final years, but, like me, she always found it hard to let things go.

It isn't as difficult a task as it might have been, because most of the furniture is to remain in the house. What has to be sorted is her clothing, which fills two double wardrobes and an enormous old chest of drawers that once belonged to her mother. It takes me days to empty those wardrobes, deciding, holding to my face her beautiful hand-knitted jumpers, breathing in her scent and sitting down on her bed to cry. Then recovering to tackle the shoes, the scarves, the costume jewellery. The quantity of stuff in her bedroom seems endless, and after a few hours of sorting it I leave, exhausted, to return another day and pick up where I left off.

I fill bags for the charity shop, and other bags with items to be thrown away. And the things I cannot part with: the hand-knits she laboured over; certain jackets and coats that still hold her scent and shape; her jewellery and perfumes; her soft cotton handkerchiefs; her wedding veil. All of them come home with me, as do the contents of her sideboard – china handed down from her mother and grandmother. For what else is to be done with the fragile cups and saucers, the beautiful old gilt-edged plates? Disposing of them is beyond me, but my own house becomes even more cluttered.

~

At forty-seven, my mother became a widow; I was twenty-one and my brother fifteen. For the last year of my father's life they had lived on a farm outside Penrith, at the foot of the Blue Mountains. I returned from New Zealand, where I'd been working, for the funeral and to help my mother prepare to move back to South Australia. I don't remember emptying those same wardrobes of my father's clothes, and I often wish now that I had kept something of his. It was straight after the funeral, and my thoughts were chaotic with grief, when during the packing-up I accidentally stumbled upon a secret.

I turned up a bundle of papers, which on closer inspection revealed that my father had been married before he married our mother. I can remember standing in their bedroom with the divorce papers in my hands, and feeling something close to panic. Never once, in all the years, had either of my parents mentioned this marriage. I hastily put the papers back where I'd found them, and kept their discovery to myself. It was the worst possible moment to raise such a subject with my mother, I saw that. But the knowledge had disturbed me, and I wanted to know who the woman was, and if there had been children. Years later I asked my aunt – my father's sister – and learned that the marriage had been brief; the wife had been unfaithful, so he'd filed for divorce. There had been no children. But the revelation, coming when it did, was a little destabilising, and for a long time afterwards I wondered uneasily what else I didn't know.

To this day, the sight of official documents stashed in dusty wardrobes or drawers stirs mild anxiety. And when I cleaned my mother's room, I hoped I wouldn't find anything worrisome.

~

Years ago, at the end of the school holidays, my brother came to see me. He had just returned from a road trip, driving with his younger daughter from Adelaide to Sydney. They had stopped near Penrith to visit the site of the farm where he and my parents had lived in the months before our father died. At my brother's last visit, sixteen years earlier, he had found the farmhouse demolished. All that had remained was a grapefruit tree in the garden, and the heavy river stones standing sentinel along the drive, some bearing vestiges of the old red paint.

This time he had found a stone he could lift, and carried it away. As he described wrestling it into the boot of his car, I guessed that retrieving this piece of his childhood had been the secret object of his journey. And then he told me that after I'd returned to New Zealand, and he and my mother were preparing to leave the farm, all the household goods they couldn't fit into the car they threw down a gully behind the house. His bicycle was among the things that had to be discarded.

He and his daughter went looking for the gully and eventually found it. The farm's old rainwater tanks had been flattened and thrown down there, too, presumably from the same point that he and my mother had flung their belongings years earlier. There was no sign of his bike, he said, only our mother's cast-iron pressure cooker, untouched, though missing its lid. He left it where it was and went to search for the spot where he last saw our father – the bedroom of the old house. It began to drizzle as he stood there with his eight-year-old and told her something about himself, and about the grandfather she had never known.

Whenever I think about my mother hurling her household goods – pots and pans and crockery she had treasured – into that gully, I feel as if a part of my mind has begun to whirl, or tilt, or spin on an invisible axis.

From this distance, her act of throwing seems like the shriek of anguish she never uttered in our presence, an act sparked by having to choose what to take and what to leave on the journey into widowhood. It distresses me that she could not afford even the small sum it would have cost to box up her possessions and ship them to Adelaide. But I am dizzied most of all because, though I was stricken by my father's death at the time, I see now that I remained oblivious to the ferocity of my mother's grief.

~

Between last Christmas and New Year I had drawn up a list of ways I could declutter our home. It covered several foolscap pages, and every morning I got up and worked at it as if it were my day job. I was taking a break from writing, so it was the perfect distraction. As I ticked off more and more things from the list, I began to feel quite pleased with myself, until I reached the task: *Sort out my clothes.* The weather was hot, and I didn't know where to start. In the end, I decided to see whether I could live with a greatly reduced number of garments before disposing of the excess. I have a small wardrobe in a spare bedroom, and my plan was to try to live out of that, and ignore the bulging cupboards in my own room.

At Big W, I bought thirty white wooden coathangers. These I put into the empty wardrobe, and carefully chose what to hang on them. It is a relief to have reduced choices about what to wear, and my plan is to have a garage sale for the rest, and then send whatever is left to the charity shops.

In the bottom of the small wardrobe are a pair of plain black trainers for walking, white plimsolls to wear with my two summer dresses, and two pairs of Doc Martens to wear with everything else. On the hangers are a couple of jackets, half-a-dozen skirts and shirts, a few linen pieces, two special-occasion dresses, and a clutch of nightdresses and Indian cotton kimonos. And that – along with a set of old gardening clothes – is really is all I need. As the weather cools, I will add jumpers, and some warmer jackets. One of the benefits of being old and mainly invisible is that no one gives a damn what you wear.

In her book *The Gentle Art of Swedish Death Cleaning*, Margareta Magnusson (who describes herself as aged between eighty and one hundred) documents the process of downsizing and decluttering after her husband's death in preparation for her own. She has many tips and tricks for whittling down possessions, from taking something of your own as a gift when someone invites you to dinner to being ruthless with things you've been given that you don't really want.

Interestingly, Magnusson suggests starting with clothes. 'Only keep those that you really feel you will wear, or if the sentimental connection with them is very strong.' She is adamant that one shouldn't start with photographs, letters or personal papers. 'If you start with them, you will definitely get stuck down memory lane, and may never get around to cleaning anything else.'

This is wise advice, and I have still not dared to approach the photographs, the boxes of letters or my own notebooks and diaries. In the case of the latter, which I can never imagine giving up while I'm still able to write, Magnusson has another useful suggestion. Find a box for the things you can't do without. On the outside, write in large letters: *Please Destroy*. Then, whoever is left to clean up when you're gone – and there will always be something to deal with – can dispose of these belongings without having to sift through them and wonder about your intentions.

In my excess wardrobe are the clothes I brought from my mother's house, and I am mustering the strength to let them go. There are small items of hers that I will keep, of course. Some days I like to wear her modest engagement ring, and it is lovely to spritz her perfume on my wrist. There are the pearls I gave her for her ninetieth birthday, which she wore at every opportunity, and her vintage brooches. But these are all I need as reminders – I don't need to curate a museum of her belongings. The hard part will be disposing of all those plates and teacups, and special-occasion dishes that have come down through the family.

I don't wish my excess belongings on anyone once I am gone, or at least not the sifting through and the endless considering. That should be for me to do, now, with enough equanimity to cull the broken and expired. I return to Magnusson for inspiration. Her recommendation is to start the death cleaning process around the age of sixty-five. I'm running five years late. There is much to do.

On the walk to the cafe, passing under the century-old plane trees, their withered leaves drift and fall around me like papery hands, or airborne starfish. The breeze tumbles them along the road with a scraping sound, a seasonal death rattle. Autumn is a kind of death cleaning, a process of making way for rest and regrowth.

Sadness is still a weight in my chest. I sense that people expect me to be getting over it. I see them thinking that my mother was ninety-five, a good innings, and I know I was lucky to have her in my life for so long. But what they don't seem to understand is that you're never ready to say goodbye to the very few people you truly love.

Extract from my garden journal, March 2021

Chapter 6

Things Fall Apart

'I'd like you to say the months of the year backwards for me,' says the nurse in the hospital's day procedures suite.

'Backwards? I'm not sure I can ...'

'Just give it a try.'

The nurse has the advantage in that she's fully clothed and on her feet, while I'm nearly naked under a flimsy robe and lying on a hospital trolley. She smiles encouragement.

'December, November, October ...' I start out well, but by the time I reach the month of April I am mentally darting backwards from January to check the correct order.

'You've just passed the test for dementia,' she says in the bright voice people adopt when speaking to children, to dogs and to old people. As she ticks off something on her sheet of questions, I can see that she expects me to be pleased. But I am not pleased, I am furious: I'm not here to be covertly tested for dementia; I'm here to discover why blood is showing up in places where there should not be blood.

The surgeon who performs my exploratory procedure is an Asian man with slender hands and a quiet smile. He comes to see me afterwards, when I'm dressed again and vaguely resemble a functioning human being.

'We found a cancer,' he says gently, and produces a report complete with colour photographs. 'You'll need surgery, but first we'll do a scan to see whether it has spread.'

~

I had been shocked to receive a positive result from my routine screening for bowel cancer. One of those kits sent to Australians between the ages of fifty and seventy-four every two years had arrived in the post; in the past my results had always been negative, which is why I let the kit linger unopened in a bathroom drawer. To give the screening program credit, when my specimen did not arrive, they sent a reminder.

No one likes doing this test, even though it is simple to perform. On consecutive days, a tiny amount of faecal matter is collected, and enclosed in a small plastic tube, which is then sent in a prepaid envelope to a pathology laboratory. Once I've dropped the package into a postbox I can usually forget about it for another couple of years, only this time a letter came to say that blood had been detected in my sample, and that a positive result requires a follow-up colonoscopy.

My GP reassured me that there could be any number of non-serious reasons for a positive reading. But on the day, in the colonoscopy suite, the examining doctor found a cancer. He estimated it had been there for about a year. Although I was told it was a slow-growing tumour, at the point of discovery there was no way of knowing whether it had already spread into lymph nodes, or indeed into any other part of my body.

In the period between being diagnosed and having the CT scan that confirmed my bowel was the primary site, I felt very alone with my body. I existed in a strange, dream-like limbo in which I would forget my situation for periods of time. But every morning, on waking, I'd remember: I have cancer! All over the world, every day, people must wake to this same bleak realisation. More than anything, it felt like a betrayal – as if the body I had lived in for a lifetime, and sometimes mistreated but mostly tended with care, had gone rogue and become my secret enemy.

I thought of the old black-and-white snapshot from my childhood. That small girl, sitting quietly on a box in the company of two cloth rabbits, looked so pure. Surely nothing ugly could ever grow inside her perfect body. Yet all these years later, a doctor has said she has a cancer. I struggled to believe it, even as I knew for certain it was true.

There was a time, perhaps when I was around eleven or twelve, when I'd try, and fail, to fall asleep at night, and in the dark I'd begin to imagine what it would be like if either of my parents died. Eventually, their loss would become so real to me that I'd begin to weep. Even as this was happening, my parents would be in the other room watching television, or fast asleep in their own bed, safe, as far as I knew. Yet the fear of their deaths was real to me in that darkened bedroom. Even now, if I close my eyes, I can place myself in the single bed; I can see dim outlines of the furniture and the curtains, and the bulk of the old upright piano against one wall. Many children must experience such fears, but whatever has triggered their anxiety recedes, until it fades away. But here's the thing:

when you live long enough, what you feared all those years ago will finally come to pass; it will become part of history. And the fear you now face in the darkness is the loss of your self.

The naturopath I consulted after my diagnosis advised me to eat deeply pigmented foods, like beetroot and berries. Also garlic, ginger, turmeric, mushrooms. She recommended sardines – Brunswick, wild-caught, in olive oil – to be eaten three times a week. Unfortunately, I have never been able to abide the sight or smell of sardines.

'Practise mindfulness and meditation every day, as well as tai chi and yoga. Walk as much as you can, and address any grief, bitterness, unforgiveness and rage.'

I had just had a novel published, and before the diagnosis I had been arranging a launch. A date had been set at the Wheatsheaf Hotel in a room prettily strung with party lights, and I was on the point of ordering catering. Even after the diagnosis it seemed as if I might still squeeze in the launch. As my publisher put it – we can have a cheer-up party before the hospital has you in its clutches. But the date set for surgery turned out to be three days before the proposed book launch, and I had to cancel.

~

The hospital has sent an appointment for a scan, and the result will determine my future – surgery, of course, but chemotherapy or no chemotherapy, radiation, prognosis. After noting it in my diary, I wash my hair and spend a long time teasing out the knots. My curly hair is halfway to my waist, and I wonder whether I will lose it; I wonder whether I should cut it shorter so that when I'm visited in my hospital bed by the medics, I will not appear to be the mad woman from the attic.

I approach the sardines via a jar of anchovies. Anchovies are not quite so repellent. I make pasta puttanesca, well laced with garlic and the little salty, slithery fillets, and manage to eat a small bowlful.

The surgeon has described the procedure as a medium to big operation. It will require three hours in theatre to cut out the section of colon containing the cancer and rejoin it using titanium staples. My recovery at home will take several months. It is a serious business and, as it's cancer, the hospital is required to deal with it within thirty days from diagnosis.

The month fills with appointments and minor medical procedures; they include an iron infusion and the scan, both of which require a cannula to be inserted into a vein. Each time, the nurse has trouble; it's as if my veins are shrinking inwards in anticipation of the onslaught. The preparations culminate in the moment I walk into the operating theatre and climb onto the table. I have been stoic, I think, throughout these worrisome weeks, but on finding myself surrounded by masked strangers, some of whom will approach with knives once I am anaesthetised, I am clammy with terror. I tell a theatre nurse that I am scared, and she reassures me that everyone in the room is there to keep me safe. Blessedly soon, the anaesthetic kicks in.

Hours later I wake up in a recovery bay, with four stab wounds and a long cut across my lower abdomen. I learn that the surgery has gone well, but it will be a week before a pathology report confirms whether the cancer has penetrated the bowel wall and spread to other places.

~

The days feel dark, even when the sun shines. I am torn between being thankful that my mother has not had to witness this frightening diagnosis and wishing with all my heart for the comfort of her presence. Cancer does strange things to the mind as well as the body, and while I know I am lucky that it was caught early, as I nurse my wounds and wait for the pathologist's report I feel halfway to dying.

    I imagine locking the gate and leaving the garden for the last time, and how without my stewardship the unpruned trees and shrubs will take more and more liberties, and the unpicked herbs will throw out seed until they choke the roses. The garden will become a wild, unruly place, the throttling ivy creeping unchecked across brick paving to explore the house. In the pond garden the fish will live for a while on mosquitoes, the fountain will slow, its filter gradually blocked by blanket weed. Then the fish will die and birds will eat them, and over the first summer the water will evaporate until there is only a scum of mud and weed at the bottom of the pond.

    The plum tree will drop its fruit in the long grass, where it will rot, and the peach tree will be stripped by rats and possums. The cumquats will fruit heavily in winter, tiny orange globes like a million lamps, unseen from the empty sitting room. The wisteria will choke the side paths. Only birds will still come, but no one will fill their water bowls on the days of ferocious heat. No one will dig worms for them, or flap their arms to scare the crows from their babies. The blackbird will visit while there is a lawn for him to forage on. He might wonder where the black-clad figure has gone, the one who would dig and weed, with him following behind. From the top of the jacaranda tree, he might pause between songs to peer into a ghost garden. He will float down and perch on the angel's head under the quince tree, king of the garden, which has always been his.

What I don't have to strain to imagine is that ever-hotter summers, and a decrease in South Australia's annual rainfall, means a future in which most of the plants I grow will be impossible to sustain. This makes me sadder than almost anything. I long to hear of real progress and innovation in the race to address climate change, but our leaders seem determined to whistle and look the other way. If they continue to ignore the need for action, then my rose bushes will one day wither and die when the precious water they need has to be diverted to the survival of trees. Knowing this makes each flowering special in the way of all things that exist on borrowed time. Where I once photographed my roses to capture and share their radiance, I now do it so that I will remember them, in case – as seems all too likely – this terrible tipping point should arrive within my lifetime.

~

During the early days of Covid, when leaving the house to shop felt dangerous, my mother pressed upon me a sheet of paper, on which she had typed Psalm 91. She knew that I could not share her beliefs, but still she insisted I carry it in my pocket whenever I went to the supermarket. The psalm, in the King James version she and I have always favoured, is one of the most reassuring texts ever written, promising protection on a biblical scale:

> Surely he shall deliver thee from the snare of the fowler, and from the noisome pestilence. He shall cover thee with his feathers, and

under his wings shalt thou trust: his truth shall be thy shield and buckler. Thou shalt not be afraid for the terror by night; nor for the arrow that flieth by day; Nor for the pestilence that walketh in darkness; nor for the destruction that wasteth at noonday. A thousand shall fall at thy side, and ten thousand at thy right hand; but it shall not come nigh thee.

To please her, I carried it in my handbag all year. But now I search it out again and keep it close; I know that if she were here, this is what she would want me to do. Because I do not have her faith, I tell myself that, if nothing else, the words are beautiful. I am managing a state of terror, where every third thought concerns death and dying; I am as helpless in my way as one of the unfledged blackbirds, and long for the protection of a pair of feathered wings.

While sitting on the veranda in the early evening I hear a great squawking of birds. I look up to see a huge dark shape glide from a distant tree; it passes out of sight, and then reappears overhead: a hawk.

All the birds are in a state of great alarm. I look for the blackbird, hoping he is safe.

Extract from my garden journal, April 2021

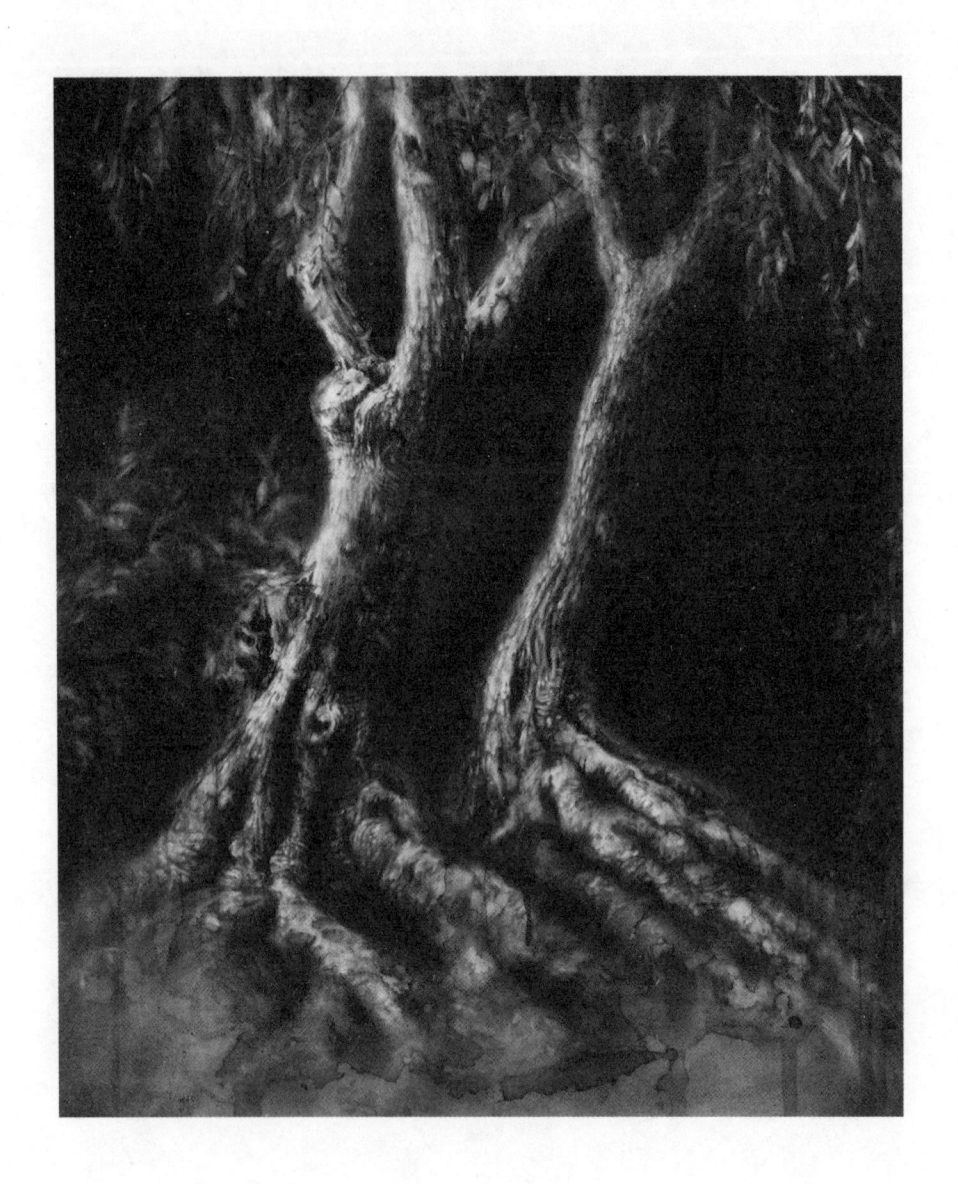

Chapter 7

Past and Future in Every Moment

At home after the surgery, I hunker down in front of the fire with a pile of books and try not to dwell on an outcome beyond the healing of my wounds. The stitches are protected under strips of surgical tape, and will dissolve. Our quiet house, with the bright leap of flames in the hearth, the sigh of logs gently subsiding and the occasional crackle and spiral of sparks, is calming medicine. Time settles during the long afternoons. I switch on the pink lamp, and my anxiety, too, begins to settle, drifting like sediment to the bottom of a glass of fresh green juice.

I am acutely aware now of everything I eat. Having seen images of the route food takes through my body I am anxious not to ingest anything that will trouble the traumatised colon. A friend tells me of the so-called Blue Zones – places in the world with unusually high numbers of healthy, active centenarians. One of these is Okinawa in southern Japan, where their long-lived population's philosophy of *kusuimun* translates as 'treat food as medicine'. Okinawans live on a mostly plant-based diet, which I also favour. In Western society we have become far removed from this concept of food as medicine; one of the small but shocking details of my hospital experience was the post-surgery meal, after three days without eating, of two highly processed sausages with fried onions, gravy and mashed potato. Processed meat products are far from ideal for a troubled bowel, so it felt as if the medical people had just saved my life and now the hospital's cooks were trying to undo their work.

It is taking a while for normal bodily functions to return, but balanced against the sometimes urgent need to rush to the bathroom is the fact that my colon is at least in working order, and I have not been burdened with the horror of a colostomy bag. This happens when it becomes necessary to attach the colon to the outside of the body via a stoma – a hole in the abdominal wall – which allows waste to leave the body. My understanding is that whether this is an outcome of the surgery depends on where in the colon the cancer is located. As in the garden, where it's good practice to pay attention to where the light falls before planting, in life, too, knowing where the light falls is important. And it seems that amid the darkness of my diagnosis, the light has fallen on where the cancer was positioned, so that I'm beyond grateful not to be dealing with the bleakness of a tube protruding from my abdomen.

Realistically, though, there is no guarantee that – down the track – I'll continue to be so lucky. Because there could be a next time, and although I try not to think about it now, while my body is still recovering, sometimes the future rears up, a giant question mark that compels me to wonder how much time is left – with or without the cancer.

The same question weighs on the character in Marion Halligan's story

'Cherubs' in which a woman who owns a large oval mirror 'garlanded with ribbons and roses, cherubs and trumpets', breaks off a cherub's foot every year on her birthday. 'She has been doing it ever since she began doing it.' Even so, some of the cherubs still retain both their fat little feet. Others have one foot, and still others are completely footless; she doesn't count them. The woman keeps the snapped-off feet in a cloisonné box, which from time to time she rattles. The question she asks herself is whether she will run out of cherubs' feet before she runs out of birthdays, or vice versa. There is a third possibility, and that is that 'there are left as many cherubs' feet as she will have years. That when they run out so will her birthdays.' The woman feels there is a secret symmetry to this that is right. While she doesn't count the remaining feet, it's a covert form of fortune-telling she's indulging in, an attempt to keep an eye on the sand trickling through the hourglass.

It is one thing to be aware that we must die, but quite another to know the when and where of it. If we knew for certain, would we be able to think about anything else? Better not to count cherubs' feet.

Knowing and not knowing is one of the defining differences between humans and animals, and yet most of us manage to hold in place some kind of barrier against the thought of our own demise. This is the opposite of the concept of memento mori (remember that you must die) proposed by the Stoic philosophers such as Seneca, who urged his followers to 'prepare our minds as if we'd come to the very end of life. Let us postpone nothing. Let us balance life's books each day. The one who puts the finishing touches on their life each day is never short of time.' The Stoics insist memento mori gives life greater meaning, and reminds us to treat each day as a gift.

Keeping death at the front of our minds in this way seems like a sensible philosophy. Because which of us doesn't want to cease frittering precious time on useless pursuits? Don't we all wish to discover greater meaning in our lives, and to wake up full of the joy of the gift of a new day? But what if we can't master the Stoic mindset?

~

Understanding what it means to age constantly raises one's relationship with time. When I was young I felt practically immortal; there seemed to be so much time and, as life stretched to infinity, old age was so distant it was pretty much irrelevant. Even so, there were rare events that shook that belief, sudden losses of schoolfriends through unexpected catastrophes or unsuspected illnesses. But even as my friends and I mourned these losses, we looked away, along our own particular pathways, squinting against the brightness that awaited us, holding intact the certainty of our own futures.

Then, in middle age, whether we measured time in minutes, hours and days or in cherubs' feet, most of us became queasily aware of a clock somewhere that would one day cease ticking. Perhaps we had experienced the first of our health scares. The losses among our peers were still not too alarming, yet not so uncommon as they had been, either. At forty-five and fifty we were on our guard: we developed exercise routines and paid closer attention to diet.

If time is a river, it only flows in one direction, and by the age of seventy most of us will have begun to wonder how far we have paddled downstream. How much further before the current sweeps us out into the vast ocean of souls who have gone before. If we were to wallow in this wondering it might induce a kind of paralysis, so that living ground to a halt long before it was time. I assume this is what ails the demographic my cousin, a psychiatric nurse, once referred to as 'the elderly depressed', although at the time she said it I was young enough to have no inkling of what she meant.

Reaching my threescore-and-ten milestone has felt at times like arriving at a delta of sorts, a scrap of ground by the wayside where one can draw breath, stop worrying about outcomes and simply delight in the small pleasures of everyday life, of which there are still many. The idea of an intermediate space between Young Old Age and Old Old Age is appealing; it evokes a sense of stillness in which time might stretch in both directions in a way that resists temporal measurements.

It is in this mood that I find solace in gardening. There is a timelessness to the routine tasks of weeding, digging, planting, and an immortal quality to knowing that many of the plants I nurture were once grown centuries earlier by monks in their physic gardens. The seeds I harvest from old medicinal herbs, such as rue, clary sage and lady's mantle, have evolved from plants that would be recognised by ancient men and women. The unbroken thread that stretches into the distant past is calming, and grounding, and gently draws my attention back to the present moment.

In a conversation about ageing and gardens with an Adelaide landscape designer, he tells me that he loves the word 'senescence'. Later, when I look it up, I find that while ageing is a progressive decline, senescence occurs throughout a lifetime, with important roles in development, as well as in wound healing. We sit together at dusk in a garden he designed almost fifty years earlier, whose owner, Bronte, is now eighty-five, while he explains the layers of earlier gardens that are present, notably in the form of an elderly pomegranate whose wizened shape has evolved into a sculptural element, and an olive tree he estimates is between 150 and 170 years old. All the stones in the garden, of which there are many, were saved from demolished railway stations by an earlier owner, who piled them underneath an enormous buddleia with the intention of doing something with them one day.

'And he never did,' says this man who describes himself only as 'Bronte's gardener'. 'But we did.'

'It's like people. We watch people senesce, and it's just part of life. We are here for that moment, we shine, and then we decline. But don't throw away the pomegranate, let it live. Like with the old olive – most people say that's past its use-by date, but I say no, it's just graciously senescing.'

I ask him whether he feels that time moves differently in a garden.

'There's a whole layer of meaning that isn't sequential. As you get older with a garden like this, you never lose the time that you've had at the beginning. You are continually going along with it as it grows. But those layers you had when you were younger, let's say fifty years ago, have added to how you sense that garden fifty years later. Because you never forget – I remember the lawn, and why we did the lawn, then we did the roses; it didn't quite work, but that's okay. It does slow time down completely.'

As a designer, his ultimate aim for a successful garden is to create mystery. 'To sit in a garden at dusk, and it feels mysterious, almost as if the previous ghosts of the garden are hanging around.'

Yet to reach even Young Old Age is to understand, perhaps for the first time, that death is not abstract, that one is now in what is often unkindly referred to as 'God's waiting room' and could be called at any moment. You might say that from the time we are born we are all waiting. And waiting is, after all, a frequent activity in daily life, one by which we avert chaos – such as when we wait at traffic lights, queue at a supermarket checkout or await our turn in a doctor's surgery.

When we wait, we are caught in an in-between space, which might be thought wasteful of precious time; it is doubtless this that makes people jump red lights or barge their way to the front of a queue. However, the French philosopher and scientist Blaise Pascal viewed these small moments in the course of a day in which we wait for something as a sign that life is worth living. If we wait, it must be assumed there is something we feel is worth waiting for.

Waiting need not be passive, and if we *live* our waiting it holds the potential for a special kind of creativity, perhaps even the 'coming into flower' described by the French writer Victor Hugo. In her essay 'Waiting on Death Row' Tamara Kohn describes 'the creative impulse that potentially blossoms in a waiting area that is off-limits to most law-abiding people'. While most of us at seventy are not contemplating the future from prison cells, we are on an existential 'death row'. Kohn suggests we can 'challenge the conditions of stasis and stagnation implicit in the term "waiting" ... with one of active making of selves and attentiveness to the present'.

In 'Waiting for Rain in the Goulburn Valley' Rosemary Robins introduces the notion of biding time. 'The activities of "biding time" are very different to those of waiting. To bide time is to remain, to wait in stillness as time passes.' This calm abiding feels close to what I imagine could happen in the space by the wayside between old age and extreme old age, or between either of those life stages and death. The elderly

Lady Slane of Sackville-West's *All Passion Spent* relishes the fact that 'For the first time in her life – no, for the first time since her marriage – she had nothing else to do. She could lie back against death and examine life. Meanwhile, the air was full of the sound of bees.'

While our lifespans appear to operate on linear time, there are other, gentler patterns, like the cyclical time that operates in nature, or in the lives of nomadic people. Nomads follow the seasons in pursuit of pasture for their animals, but as they grow older they take on tasks that require less movement, and turn their attentions to preparations for the next life. Lady Slane does her lying back against death in a house in Hampstead with a lovely garden, which she has long coveted. Gardens allow us to observe complete life cycles in both plants and animals, and the cycles return with reassuring regularity.

In Nathaniel Hawthorne's short story 'The Haunted Mind' there is a wonderfully precise description of the pleasure of waking from sleep when there are hours of darkness still ahead – of occupying the 'intermediate space' by the wayside, in which time lingers – before his protagonist gloomily declares, 'In the depths of every heart there is a tomb and a dungeon'. It seems that, after all, we humans are haunted – unless we build that wall against knowing, and even then, which wall in history has ever successfully excluded the unwanted?

Ten years after the death of the feted Argentine writer Jorge Luis Borges, American writer Susan Sontag wrote an open letter to him that contained this observation: 'You had a sense of time that was different from other people's. The ordinary ideas of past, present and future seemed banal under your gaze. You liked to say that every moment of time contains the past and the future ...' Borges himself had written of time as a river: 'Time is the substance I am made of. Time is a river which sweeps me along, but I am the river; it is a tiger which destroys me, but I am the tiger; it is a fire which consumes me, but I am the fire.'

If time is a tiger which destroys me, and if I am the tiger, if it is a fire which consumes me and I am the fire, am I guilty of destroying what remains of my life? In the anticipation of suffering, we suffer twice. I may worry whether the cancer that's been removed will return, but for all I know I may live half as long again as I've already lived. That would put me at 105, which is unlikely though not impossible. Yet it is rare enough that I imagine such longevity bringing with it the profound loneliness that must engulf any creature that finds itself the last of its kind. If everyone I have loved has gone, would I wish to stay?

Having tested us with the vision of the tomb and the dungeon, Hawthorne returns in the end to the beauty and strangeness to be found in 'the wilderness of sleep'. A distant clock marks the start of 'a temporary death'. For the remaining hours of the night, our spirit will stray 'like a free citizen among the people of a shadowy world, beholding strange sights, yet without wonder or dismay. So calm, perhaps, will be the final change – so undisturbed, as if among familiar things, the entrance of the soul to its eternal home'.

Closing the gap between death and sleep sounds like the wishful inscription found on many a tombstone: *Her end was Peace*. Yet it also evokes an enviable passing, unlike the visions of tortured struggles that haunt us in the wee small hours. Modern medicine, too, works to close the gap, with its morphine pumps and discreet doses of anti-anxiety drugs for the dying.

In Australian culture, death and dying remain as shrouded in mystery as ever, despite happening all around us every day of the week. Some of us lose ourselves in our art and writing. Some build walls against knowing, some seek refuge in religion, while others seek to erase the knowing with drugs and alcohol, or a life so crammed with activity that there is no time to think. Some brave souls strive to settle into the Stoic mindset, to face the fact of death and live each day as if it were their last.

In *Mrs Dalloway*, Virginia Woolf writes: 'The compensation of growing old [is] that the passions remain as strong as ever, but one has gained – at last! – the power which adds the supreme flavour to existence – the power of taking hold of experience, of turning it around, slowly, in the light.'

Straining after the past and peering fearfully towards the future is likely to result in a mind so agitated it is incapable of performing this slow turning. So it is up to each of us to vanquish our inner tiger, to extinguish our damaging fire, or risk being swept past the place by the wayside where, like Lady Slane, we can lie back against death and examine life. Then, if we are lucky, we may find ourselves biding time in an intense and joyful present, and for all we know this is the moment in a life where, in this slow turning, the meaning of it all is at last made clear.

The shadow patterns in the garden have shifted as the autumn sun sets a new course. Light slants deeper into the veranda and heats the tiles, where I sit soaking in the warmth. There is an almost narcotic-like drowsiness about these still afternoons, and even the bees move more slowly. Spiders have been busy, and the fine filaments of their webs sway with the slightest breath of air. Magpies carol madly. Rose leaves glint, and the quince trees are laden.

Autumn, even early on, has a richness and an intensity. The roses that flower now are not so numerous, nor so large, but the colour of their buds and petals is more concentrated than in spring. Parrots visit the garden in pairs. I watch them walking along the top of the brush fence with their quaint, faintly comic gait. From there they drift into the fig tree, having cannily spied the last of the fruit. Autumn is all about plenty, and the last of plenty, and the cycle of death and regeneration.

Extract from my garden journal, April 2021

Chapter 8

The Possibility of Radiance

Ageist thought patterns and reactions are so embedded in Australian culture that even educated people, people who otherwise insist on political correctness, will open their mouths and deliver a hurtful, hateful judgement. I'm remembering the time, sitting on the grass at a writers' festival with a group of other women writers of whom I was the oldest. We were fellow graduates from a postgraduate creative writing course, some of us just beginning to be published; I knew the generational difference made parts of my life inaccessible to them, as parts of their lives would remain mysterious to me.

That afternoon, with literary conversations buzzing all around, I remarked in passing that I was thinking of colouring my hair with henna. That rich and blazing plant-based red had once been my signature shade, but what with study, family and moving countries, the process of sourcing, mixing up and applying the henna had all come to seem too messy, too difficult.

So I had let my colour fade; I had allowed a succession of hairdressers to cover my grey hairs with chemical dyes, at ridiculous expense.

Immediately, one of the women blurted: 'Oh, I wouldn't. Not at your age!'

My thoughts seemed to skid to a halt. I was fifty-nine: too old to need anyone's approval or permission. Lost for a response, I remained silent. Out of all of us, this woman was the one who was always bleaching or dyeing or doing something to her hair, in the process often leaving it visibly damaged. My memory of that moment is that she realised what she had said was offensive, and tried to retrieve it by disparaging the older women with hennaed hair who regularly fill seats at the festival. However, a second ageist comment could not defuse the first.

Going further back, during the demanding MA year that would eventually result in my first published novel, I was paying the household bills by freelancing – words and pictures – for a local glossy lifestyle magazine. The editor had sent me to a country race meeting with instructions to take plenty of pictures of racegoers for the social pages. At the end of a long hot afternoon, filling time while waiting for the bus to take me back to Adelaide, I gathered a few last shots as people clambered into hired stretch limos.

Two suited-up young men were lounging in the back seat of one of these vehicles. I leaned in the open door and asked if they'd like to have their photographs taken for the social pages, and I named the magazine. They beamed obligingly; I snapped the picture, recorded their names, and turned away. And then I heard one of them say in a sniggering undertone: 'Why the hell are [name of the magazine] getting old grannies to do this work?'

I was checking their image on my digital camera, making sure the exposure was good, the framing right.

'Shhh!' hissed the friend.

I was a fifty-four-year-old woman at the end of a long working day: I was not going to put up with this. My vengeful thumb moved to delete their image. Of course, I should have turned to that arrogant boyo and asked whether he had a grandmother and, if he did, how he would feel if someone insulted her the way he had just insulted me. But I couldn't face him because my eyes had filled with tears. Walking away, I blamed my loss of control on menopause. But it wasn't that, it was the shame women are made to feel simply for having lived a certain number of years.

Both men and women suffer from the social erasing of the old, but it is worse for women. The value placed on feminine beauty means that older women often find themselves at the terrible nexus of sexism and ageism.

In 1972, in 'The Double Standard of Aging', Susan Sontag identified the oppressive belief that men are enhanced by age while women are progressively destroyed. 'Competing for a job,' writes Sontag, 'her chances often partly depend on being the "right age", and if hers isn't right, she will lie if she thinks she can get away with it.' A woman's age, Sontag insists, is 'something of a dirty secret'.

It often seems as if not much has changed since 1972. Bill Shorten once admitted that his mother Ann, having qualified as a barrister at fifty-three, found, in Bill's words, that 'sometimes, you're just too old, and you shouldn't be too old, but she discovered the discrimination against older women'.

Sex-ageism is not merely demoralising, but has the potential to affect women's ability to survive. If we are not to be allowed to continue to work even though we are fit for it, if we have always been paid less than our male colleagues, if we have given years of our lives to the unpaid labour of child rearing, if we have insufficient super (or no super at all), what is to become of us in our sixties, seventies and eighties? Are we to swell the ranks of the new demographic of homeless older women?

In *At Seventy: A Journal*, May Sarton writes, 'This is the best time of my life. I love being old.' She goes on to explain that she does not feel old at all, 'not as much a survivor as a person still on her way', and she speculates that perhaps real old age will only begin when you find yourself looking back rather than forward. Sarton's journals are rightly celebrated, and are a cache of gold well worth digging to find. For together with Doris Lessing, May Sarton is one of the few women writers who have not shied away from writing about age and ageing. The shocking scarcity of older women in fiction, which has left me with a sense of marching forward in the dark, is balanced by the steadying beam of their work – especially Sarton's, for the light she sheds is age-affirming, ever hopeful, an antidote to the 'state of decline' narrative.

For example, when asked why she thought it was good to be old, Sarton replied: 'Because I am more myself than I have ever been. There is less conflict. I am happier, more balanced, and more powerful.' She amended this to 'I am better able to use my powers'. And Sarton continued to use those powers, writing *At Eighty-Two: A Journal*. Although it was published under that title, her preferred name for it was *Kairos*, after 'a Greek word meaning a unique time in a person's life and an opportunity for change'.

This question of how to be, as we move from middle age into old age, is a lot like the dilemma of the teenage self. Back then it was the childish body transforming to adulthood, and although that destination was where most of us wished to be, the unfamiliarity of the changed self, and the pressures of fashion, popular culture and one's peers, often made the transition awkward and painful.

While the destination of Old is not where most of us wish to be, if we live long enough we will have no choice. If there is any advantage to this passage, it must be the freedom, and the power described by May Sarton, to be more ourselves than we have ever been. Yet how many of us know ourselves well enough to be 'more'?

Lately I have been taking inspiration from the musician, artist and poet Patti Smith. Now pushing deep into her seventies, Patti is a creative force; she still performs with her band. Smith describes herself as 'always evolving', but not changing because of any outside pressure. Never one to conform to expectations of feminine beauty, or of how a woman should appear on a stage, Smith appears to be a completely authentic version of her younger self, only older.

Realising this authentic self is the task old age sets us, but how is it to be done? How are we to tell what the authentic self is? In the preface to *The Diaries of Jane Somers* Doris Lessing – who initially submitted the two novels in this volume using a pseudonym – explains that by writing under another name she wanted 'to get free of that cage of associations and labels that every established writer has to learn to live inside'. She also wanted to 'cheer up young writers, who often have such a hard time of it'.

Interestingly, both the novels in Lessing's publishing experiment deal with women and age. The first, *The Diary of a Good Neighbour*, evokes the unforgettable Maudie Fowler, who in her nineties remains so fiercely independent that she will not consider moving from the dauntingly uncomfortable rooms she inhabits, or even having helpers. "'With your own place,' Maudie says, 'you've got everything. Without it, you are a dog. You are nothing.'"

In England, Doris Lessing's publishers, Jonathan Cape and Granada, rejected *The Diary of a Good Neighbour*, with Granada saying it was 'too depressing' to publish. It was then accepted by Michael Joseph, whose editors said it reminded them of Doris Lessing. When it was acquired by Lessing's French publisher, he rang her to ask if she had helped Jane Somers, because Somers reminded him so much of her.

The perceptiveness of these publishers made Lessing question what it was they had recognised. She had deliberately made Jane Somers's style different from her own, and felt that each of her novels had a characteristic tone of voice, a style peculiar to itself. Lessing reasoned that 'behind this must sound another note, independent of style. What is this underlying tone, or voice, and where does it originate in the author? It seems to me we are listening to, responding to, the essence of a writer here, a groundnote.'

I am fascinated by this concept of the groundnote as it relates to writing, and in whether or not one can recognise it in one's own work. I am reminded of those black-and-white films we once watched on television that were set on board a submarine; the only soundtrack was the persistent *bleep* of the sonar. Often the act of writing itself is like being one of the submarine's crew – tensed within the finite oxygen supply of a tiny lit capsule, pushing on through darkness under crushing force. I can still picture those submariners: sweating, silent, while the vessel shook and water trickled dangerously, and the periscope was cranked up to scan the surface.

Aside from writing, Doris Lessing's experiment easily relates to the dilemmas of ageing, for older women, too, suffer the 'cage of associations and labels'. It is good to be reminded that, whatever style we adopt, or imagine we possess, there is, underneath, the groundnote of the true self.

Patti Smith writes in *M Train*:

As a child I thought I would never grow up, that I could will it so. And then I realized, quite recently, that I had crossed some line, unconsciously cloaked in the truth of my chronology. How did we get so damn old? I say to my joints, my iron-coloured hair.

Yet, Smith continues: 'If we walk the victim, we're perceived as the victim. And if we enter ... glowing and receptive ... if we maintain our radiance and enter a situation with radiance, often radiance will come our way.'

Understanding our groundnote must surely release us into our power. Hearing it, will we not become comfortable, even radiant, in our own skins? I am visualising a state of being that has nothing to do with the positive ageing or active ageing campaigns directed towards the elderly. Those campaigns could be termed passive-aggressive, for their subtext is that ageing is bad. And in denying age its due dignity, in promoting a fantasy in which old people do not appear to age at all, they set the scene for many levels of failure.

So how are we to hear this groundnote? It might be a case of careful and consistent listening. It must be different for everyone. Perhaps the transition is less about growing old and more about growing up. When I think about this what comes to mind is the Michelle Shocked song

'When I Grow Up', with its implication of a genuine desire to experience being an old woman. If there are stages we must pass through, the first stage might be the cessation of denial.

The feminist writer Betty Friedan admits that in her fifties she 'didn't even want to think about age'; she was locked in denial. But eventually she 'began to recognize some new dimension of personhood, some strength or quality of being in people who had crossed the chasm of age – and kept on going and growing'.

In her book *The Feminine Mystique*, Friedan, at thirty-five, had refused to let women be defined as sex objects, and in *The Fountain of Age*, her book on age, she refuses to let women or men over sixty-five be defined as objects of 'care', or old age be defined as a sickness to be cured.

Feminism has fought hard for women's rights, but despite some of the movement's leaders researching exhaustively and writing about women and ageing, ageism persists. The last of the undesirable 'isms' to ever be mentioned, it is normalised in Australian culture. Old women remain the butt of jokes and are some of society's most marginalised people.

Feminists have typically addressed matters affecting younger women. This reflects the age of the women involved in the battles for equal pay, paid maternity leave and the calling-out of sexual harassment. Sadly, when it comes to old women, even younger women do not see them. The result is mutual deprivation: old women have no opportunity to contribute their experience and wisdom, and young women have no role models to show them how to manage their own inevitable ageing.

One thing that gives me hope this will change is the grey-hair movement on Instagram. Candid posts celebrating the many and varied beauties of naturally greying hair could both encourage the hairdressing industry to find ways to ease the transition and help recalibrate perceptions of female beauty.

I was pleased to discover an Australian novel in which the main characters are all women in their seventies. Charlotte Wood's *The Weekend* goes against the grain of decades of published fiction, with just a few notable exceptions.

Wood's literary currency means the book has been widely read, and at literary festivals it sparked conversations about ageing, and especially about what it means for women. In the novel, the elderly actress Adele has a moment when she feels 'on the edge of discovering something very important – about living, about the age beyond youth and love, about this great secret time of a person's life'. Perhaps Adele is about to discover her *kairos*.

Liz Byrski is another Australian writer who has identified the absence of old people, especially old women, in fiction, and has set herself the task of addressing it. In her novels she makes a point of showing old women using computers and mobile phones, busting the stereotype of elders baffled by technology. In her slender book *Getting On: Some Thoughts on Women and Ageing* Byrski insists we challenge the public perception of ageing and change it to 'a positive conversation in which the phrase "the fight against ageing" is banned and the use of "anti-ageing" as a descriptor for any product is greeted with derision'. She goes on to suggest how as individuals we should 'start seeing old people': we should strive to put aside our blindness, denial and fear, and focus instead on the richness and value of the lives old people are still living.

The negativity around ageing, the elitism of youth, means there are few older role models to encourage our young people. This has the effect of leaving them marooned, unable to imagine a way forward, beyond middle age – and further on into the kind of old age that, if they are lucky enough to reach it, they might be willing, even proud, to live.

In *The Element of Lavishness: Letters of Sylvia Townsend Warner and William Maxwell,* Maxwell writes to Warner – in the last of his letters to her before she died – of his father-in-law, who had just turned ninety-two. He had 'always been a good letter writer but his letters have recently taken on a kind of radiance, as if he had stopped taking any ordinary part in life, stopped worrying'. Maxwell goes on to explain that he means worrying about 'the outcome of things'. Instead, it seems the old man was simply looking around him with delight 'at the way everything is'.

Susan Sontag, while describing old age as a 'genuine ordeal', maintained it was mainly 'an ordeal of the imagination'. I don't believe she was underestimating the physical tests and challenges age brings, but rather acknowledging that nothing about it is so testing as being looked through, looked past, being patronised, being treated by others as diminished or worthless.

By continuing to denigrate old age we are contributing to this ordeal, condemning young folk to 'walk the victim', denying them, and ourselves, the possibility of *kairos*: the possibility of radiance.

Part III
Winter

Never are voices so beautiful as on a winter's evening, when dusk almost hides the body, and they seem to issue from nothingness with a note of intimacy seldom heard by day.

Night and Day, Virginia Woolf

Chapter 9

When Enough Is Enough

Choosing voluntary assisted dying

Not long ago, on a morning when the house was quiet and the garden was flooded with clear winter light, I opened an email from a friend to learn that she had chosen to access voluntary assisted dying to end her life. She wrote that she was feeling quite accepting, and that she had met with the palliative care team to talk about her end-of-life care and where that should happen.

By the time I had read to the end of her email I was weeping. My friend, an acclaimed poet, had just published a memoir and a book of poetry. She was still in her fifties; one had imagined a sparkling body of work to come, and then there was her family – elderly parents on the far side of the world, and at home, her partner and their three children.

I had known she had cancer, and that she'd undergone surgeries and rounds of chemotherapy. But the last time I had seen her she'd been on a new treatment regime and had assured me it seemed to be working. After that, she went quiet. Her silence should have alerted me, but instead I chose to believe that, as the deeply private person she was, she was just withdrawing into her home and family to allow herself the best possible chance to heal.

~

As human beings we all have a terminal diagnosis, it's just that we haven't as yet been given a timeframe. Living a more or less functional life requires us to perform a delicate balancing act between knowing and not knowing we will die. Fear of extinction is the first of the five fears that are said to drive us; it's at the top of a list that includes mutilation, loss of autonomy, separation and ego death. The longer one lives, each of these feared conditions becomes less of an abstract possibility and more of a likelihood, and when I consider that list in the context of old age I am both startled and humbled by the grace with which old people bear up.

Our understanding of death develops gradually, from a first dim awareness between the ages of three through to five, when the deaths of birds and pet animals prompt our first encounter with the word 'dead'. Small children cannot grasp theoretical concepts such as 'forever', so if someone they know has died most will expect the person to return. Between the ages of five and seven, we begin to realise that all living things eventually die, and that death is irreversible. From nine, and onwards through adolescence, we understand that death is not only irreversible but that we, too, will one day die.

Nearly everyone fears death, and that fear is the focus of terror management theory, a concept developed by social psychologists Jeff Greenberg, Sheldon Solomon and Tom Pyszczynski. Their work was based on that of cultural anthropologist Ernest Becker, who in *The Denial of Death* wrote: 'The knowledge of death is reflective and conceptual, and animals are spared it. They live and they disappear with the same thoughtlessness: a few minutes of fear, a few seconds of anguish, and it is over. But to live a whole lifetime with the fate of death haunting one's dreams and even the most sun-filled days – that's something else.'

Terror management theory is an anxiety-buffering system that helps humans manage their fear of dying. Our awareness of death requires defensive manoeuvres that help us think of it as something we don't need to worry about until some indefinite time in the distant future.

In her book *The Museum of Words*, Australian writer Georgia Blain documents her experience of being diagnosed at fifty-one with a Stage 4 brain cancer:

> Everything came down to the same pinprick piercing the page: We are all dying. We all should be living life appreciating the beauty of the ordinary. But so often we don't. And this is the eternal human paradox; the only way we can cope with our mortality is to ignore it, to live as though we have all the time in the world.

In *The Denial of Death*, Becker confirms this human need. 'Beyond a given point man is not helped by more "knowing", but only by living and doing in a partly self-forgetful way.'

The focus of religions has often helped in this objective: how to live while bearing the knowledge of the end of life. But religious faith is no longer so widespread, at least in Western culture. This leaves many of us to juggle an end-of-life experience without the comforting prospect of a better life beyond the one we know.

Blain describes the loneliness she felt, post diagnosis. 'The nature of a life-threatening disease makes you separate out from other people, and you are alone with it.' She revealed that at times she was 'awash with sorrow and grieving', but there were also moments when life seemed to have an intensity she had never felt before. 'I was leaving the world, crossing to the other side, never really being able to join the living again.'

On re-reading my friend's email, in which she was saying goodbye, I sensed that she, too, felt alone and separate, despite being surrounded by a loving, grieving family. But she had seized control of the illness she'd been told would destroy her, and with a poet's instinct for finding pulse-points she had drilled down beyond terror management to grasp the quick of life and assert her ownership. In leaving the world at a day and time of her choosing, it struck me that she had engaged the same freewheeling spirit and raw courage that moves a creatively gifted mind.

Becker describes how the fear of death drives humans to seek a feeling of heroic value, and to create something of lasting worth that will 'outlive and outshine death and decay'. 'Society itself is a codified hero system, which means that society everywhere is a living myth of the significance of human life, a defiant creation of meaning.'

Terror of death is also at the root of our sense of self-preservation. This sets choosing to die in opposition to such fundamentally strong, conscious and unconscious forces that from the outside it is almost impossible to comprehend such a decision.

In *The View in Winter: Reflections on Old Age*, British writer Ronald Blythe observes, 'It is as though one needs a special strength to die, and not a final weakness.' Becker agrees, quoting American palaeontologist Nathaniel Shaler: 'We admire most the courage to face death; we give such valor our highest and most constant adoration; it moves us deeply in our hearts because we have doubts about how brave we ourselves would be.'

Certainly, when I learned of my friend's decision to access assisted dying, I felt it demonstrated an almost super-human strength and courage, a courage I could not imagine ever possessing.

~

After seventeen attempts since 1993, the Voluntary Assisted Dying Act was finally passed by the South Australian Parliament on 24 June 2021 and became available from 31 January 2023. All states in Australia have now passed a Voluntary Assisted Dying (VAD) law, allowing VAD as an end-of-life choice.

To be eligible for assisted dying, a patient must be assessed by two doctors who have been registered and trained to support the voluntary assisted dying process. To fit the criteria, you must be eighteen or older, and an Australian citizen or permanent resident. In South Australia you must have lived in the state for at least twelve months at the time of making your first request. You must have been diagnosed with a disease, illness or medical condition that is incurable, that is advanced and progressive, and that will cause death within six months, or twelve months if neurodegenerative, such as motor neurone disease. People suffering from mental illness or disability without also having a medical condition that meets the criteria are not considered eligible.

Only the patient can start a conversation about voluntary assisted dying with a health practitioner. The Act prevents health professionals from raising the topic.

~

I have now been told that my own surgery caught the cancer before it spread, and that I will not need chemotherapy, only monitoring going forward. I wept with relief when the news came. But I've not yet shaken off the terror of those days while I waited to learn what would come next, and I will never again feel quite so sure of my own body.

What is to be done with terror, especially the terror of choosing the moment of one's own death? With age, I've learned that ignorance and a vivid imagination are my worst enemies, and the only thing to do when something frightens me is to seek information.

So I contact someone who has an important role with patients who choose voluntary assisted dying. Lauren is the lead pharmacist tasked with providing the medications here in South Australia, and from her I learn that unless you are unable to hold a glass and drink through a straw, or if you are unable to absorb medication from your gut into your bloodstream – meaning that you can't take medicines orally – the medication will be self-administered. It's only if you are unable to do either of those things that you qualify for a practitioner administration, and the majority of people who access VAD administer the medication themselves, by mouth.

The drug is delivered as a powder that is mixed with a liquid before use. The dose is sufficient to sedate the person, and they fall asleep within a couple of minutes. For most people, when it's taken orally, death will occur within thirty minutes to an hour. If someone has a weak heart, or weak lungs, it might be faster. Occasionally people respond differently, in which case it might take several hours during which they'll go into a deep sleep, and their breaths will come further and further apart. When the drug is administered intravenously by a practitioner it can work faster – perhaps ten to fifteen minutes.

Legislation requires that on dispensing or supplying medication, a pharmacist must provide a certain amount of information. Because of the nature of the drug, this has to be delivered verbally, in person.

'We go into people's homes,' Lauren says, 'and we check whether we're comfortable with supplying it, we check the ID. We check that they are still able to swallow and ensure that someone is able to make up the suspension.'

The medication arrives in a small jar with the pre-measured amount of the drug, along with a 30ml bottle of the mixing agent. It's a simple matter of tipping the contents of the bottle into the jar, putting the lid back on and giving it a shake. People who are really unwell might not be able to manage that, but Lauren notes that some people are very determined to do it themselves and don't want anybody else to be the one to prepare it.

'We check that they understand what will happen if they take the medication. We ask people to tell us in their own words what will happen, and then we ask them – knowing that taking this medication will result in death – whether they want us to supply it to them. If they say, "Not today", that's fine. But if they say yes, then we will get the kit and hand it over.' The pharmacist will spend about an hour with people, giving them time to ask questions. Lauren says, 'Sometimes it's just the patient and their contact person, or it can be a big crowd of people. It's quite variable.'

When I ask what the mood is like at this moment of handing over the means to end a life, Lauren says, 'Often people feel relieved, and you get a definite sense of their relief. But at times it can be very emotional. Sometimes it's almost like the grief process starts there, and not just for the person. It hits everybody differently.'

Quietly, Lauren stresses what I already know – that nobody wants to die, and nobody is accessing VAD because they want to die. They're just at different levels of acceptance of the inevitability of death, and there are different levels of fear around what that could look like.

'It's as individual as people are,' Lauren says. 'But you can see that you are giving some degree of power back to someone who was otherwise powerless. And even if it's just having the medication and putting it in the cupboard and never even looking at it again, that's enough for some people.'

Some choose to go out in a celebratory style. They'll organise a living wake, with friends and family having drinks and nibbles. Other people plan for worst-case scenarios and may not intend to use the medication until a certain stage of their disease is reached. Others will have a date in mind and are planning towards that. A percentage of people never use the medication.

I ask whether this process is draining for the attending pharmacist.

'It's surprisingly uplifting, because you can see relief and power and choice. But I've never been in a job where you self-reflect so much. It does make you aware of your own life and relationships.'

Everyone the pharmacists visit is already dying; that is the path they are on.

'Nothing's changing the destination. It's just that they're choosing to get there a little bit faster.'

The medication tastes bitter, which somehow seems fitting. Lauren says they try to prepare people for that, and advise them to drink it quickly, and to have something handy to drink before and after. People who drink alcohol might see it as a ceremonial moment, with a special whisky or a glass of champagne.

'Unfortunately, with bitter flavours, you can't really mask it, so if we add syrups or flavourings, it doesn't do much for the taste and it just makes the volume bigger. It's about the volume of a shot, 30ml, so one big mouthful. It's very unlikely that they're not going to have swallowed enough for it to take effect.'

For health practitioners with a person-centred approach, VAD can be seen as a natural progression of helping to relieve suffering in a way that is acceptable to the patient and in alignment with their values and choices. It can be argued that it is not so very different from when someone decides to hasten their own end by refusing treatment.

Accepting that death is not a failure of the health system appears to be one of the main challenges in getting medical practitioner participation, that and attitudes towards death in health communities. Although VAD is now legal in all states, it exists amid a strong sense of taboo and an ongoing silence. Ensuring that communities are better informed might help overcome that, as well as provide support for people who are asked to be the patient's contact person.

VAD is not the same as suicide but, as with suicide, the grief and loss aren't felt only by the person experiencing the disease; they take a toll on the people around them. When I ask Lauren to define for me the difference between VAD and suicide, she is clear.

'The difference between VAD and suicide is that when someone commits suicide it's treated as an unnatural death, which has a whole host of implications. The person has to act completely alone, so that none of their loved ones are implicated. The place of death is treated as a crime scene and all that goes with that. There is a coronial investigation and autopsy. It impacts life insurance and probity. Basically, there are all sorts of factors that cause distress, far beyond the ending of a life.'

With voluntary assisted dying, the experience is very different. The person is able to be open with their plans and share their last moments, supported by their loved ones. Their body can be cared for in accordance with their customs. The coroner is notified, but on the death certificate the cause of death is given as the underlying condition. Tick boxes allow the doctor to say whether they know that the person had access to VAD, and whether they took the medication. While this provides an indication to Births Deaths and Marriages, and a notification to the coroner, it doesn't appear on the death certificate sent to the family, so their confidentiality is protected.

~

In the JM Coetzee short story 'As a Woman Grows Older', seventy-two-year-old Elizabeth Costello tells her daughter, 'There is one thing the old are better at than the young, and that is dying. It behooves the old (what a quaint word!) to die well, to show those who follow what a good death can be.'

It seems that a good death requires enormous courage, and I am filled with admiration for people like my friend who take control of a desperate situation and make it play out on their own terms. Although for the moment it seems I myself might be out of the woods, I know there could be a return, or a development in some other area. After all, I am roughly the same age as Elizabeth Costello, an age where so many things can go wrong.

This is the problem humans face: what to do about the fear of dying while keeping on living. According to terror management theory 'death anxiety drives people to ... believe that they play an important role in a meaningful world'. People strive to insulate themselves from a deep fear of living an insignificant life that is destined to be erased by death. I imagine this is one of the drivers of my desire to write, to publish, to leave something behind, however obscure.

The trouble with death is that its effect ripples outwards from the one who is dying to family, friends and friends of friends and family. From the moment I learned the time and date of my friend's death I could think of nothing else. Every clock in the world was ticking towards it.

On the appointed morning, I woke to fog. A soft, moist mist enveloped the entire city; it was like a blessing bestowed, and I couldn't help but feel it had come because of my friend – for years she had pined for the weather of her native Scotland. I hoped she would have a glimpse of it, that it would comfort her, and finally enfold her in its softness. The indistinct outlines of everything made the morning bearable for me, but not, I imagine, for my friend, for her husband and their three grieving bairns.

Two months after her death, her friends gathered for a memorial event at the Wheatsheaf Hotel, where she had often taken part in poetry readings. It was an emotional evening, interspersed with audio recordings of her reading some of her own poems. The last poem she wrote was included in an obituary in the online publication where she had been an arts reviewer. Perhaps it is the first time a poet has addressed this particular form of dying in a poem.

Unbearable lightness
by Alison Flett

>Old self that once was dot, was free-range
>cells. What whispered magic spun me
>from your coiled chains, made blue veins
>and solid thump of heart? Plump meat, bone,
>breath sewn through with darts of thought?
>How came I into this? And how to reconcile return?
>To turn away from touch of skin
>on skin, from sound of song? To leave behind
>the blush of evening sky, the rush of waves
>on rock? How to enter once again the empty
>realm of naught? Old self, guide me home,
>ballasted by joy of this. Let it be enough
>to once have been.

Most poignantly, on a 'memory' that popped up on my Facebook page some months after her passing, I found that she had commented about a project we'd been planning together that had never quite come to fruition: maybe we'd get it together when we had more time.

Out walking this morning, I found a dead male blackbird at the corner of my street. Ants had begun to explore, but he was still intact. It was impossible to know what had happened, but blackbirds are low-flying, and I suspected a mistimed daredevil swoop through traffic. I covered him with my handkerchief, then lifted him and carried him home. He weighed nothing, his little body emptied of song, drawn in on himself.

At home, I scooped out the earth under one of the apple trees and lined it with the papery leaves from the plane trees that do not break down in winter. They looked like hands circled to receive him, as I gently laid him in and covered him with more leaves. Reluctantly, I filled his grave with sweet, crumbly composted soil. From now on this will be the blackbird's corner, between the Rokewood apple tree and the Granny Smith.

It is a beautiful morning. Cold but clear, with a kick of warmth in the sun. Later, there will be little puffy clouds, but for now the pale sky is pure and empty, emptier again for the loss of even this one small unnamed bird.

Extract from my garden journal, July 2021

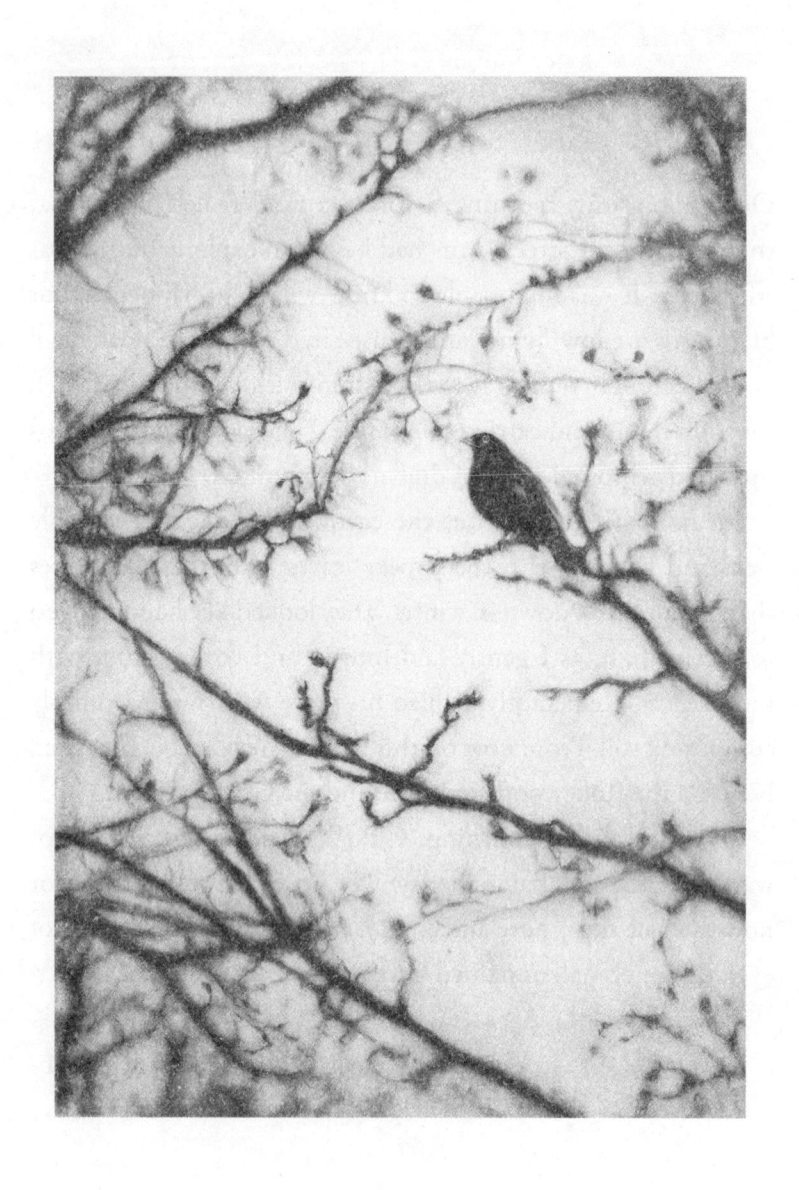

Chapter 10

Saying Goodbye

There is a last time for everything, and sometimes we know it and sometimes we don't. Of the two, not knowing can be far kinder; for example, on the Friday afternoon in January when I picked up my mother from her house to take her to ours for the weekend, she had no inkling, nor did I, that she was leaving her home for the last time. If she had somehow been made aware of it, it would have caused profound distress – she had lived in the old house as a child, and again since she moved back to Adelaide in 1972. It was where she felt happiest. As it was, leaving it on a Friday afternoon was simply part of our weekly routine. We spent our weekends together, and then on a Monday morning I would drive her home, so when she closed the front door that day it was with the expectation of returning.

The last time I saw my father was on a winter's day in Sydney, with a sharp wind swirling dust and stirring rubbish in the soiled alleyways around Kings Cross. I was leaving for New Zealand in a week, and he'd driven in from Penrith to see me. We stood on the broken concrete of the forecourt outside the flats where I had been living to say goodbye. I don't remember what I wore, but he was in his old bottle-green cable-knit jumper, V-necked and unravelling in a hole at one elbow.

He hugged me. 'I love you, darling,' he said.

There was no way of knowing then that these would be his last words to me. He was forty-nine, and although he had recently been ill, I believed he had recovered. As he drove away towards the Blue Mountains, with my cat crouched on the back seat of his old Fairlane, I was certain he still had a lot more of his life to live.

My mother's great-grandson was seventeen when she died, a young man with whom she'd shared a close and loving relationship. Of all of us, he never took it for granted that he would see her again. Perhaps he is an old soul in a young body, but whenever she left us to go home, he would insist on sitting with her and hugging her and reminding her of how much he loved her. In the hospital, he stayed beside her during her last night, mature beyond his years in the way he responded in this crisis. Of all of us, he was, I felt, the only one who had not left his goodbyes too late; he'd said them, over and over, every time they parted.

I've been raised to be casual about goodbyes with those I love. It has never struck me more than when I've made the long journey interstate to visit my surviving aunts, one of whom is elderly, while the other, at ninety-six, has entered old old age. They look forward to my visits, and we enjoy spending time together, but when it is time for me to leave, they never drag out the parting. At my last trip, just before Christmas, my eldest aunt had recently been in hospital with heart trouble. Now completely blind, she was much frailer than at my last visit, but still she walked to the gate with us.

She and I have always been close, and I have often referred to her as my second mother. Just as well I have a spare, I told her, when I rang to break the news that my mother had died. At my last visit, even though it must have crossed her mind, as it crossed mine, that there was every chance we would not meet again, after a fierce, brief hug, she turned and walked smartly back to the house. Even before she went blind, it was her habit to part this way, abruptly, with no backward glances. Although I'm pretty sure my aunt has never read the memoir *West with the Night* by Kenyan aviator and adventurer Beryl Markham, I know she'd agree with her thoughts on leaving. 'If you must leave a place that you have lived in and loved and where all your yesteryears are buried deep, leave it in any way except a slow way, leave it the fastest way you can.'

The young man who adored my mother has taught me not to leave what we wish to say until the eulogies at the funeral. Tell them each time we meet and part that they are precious. It's the only way we can be certain that they know.

As I walk to the cafe for my morning coffee, the light under the leafless plane trees is so dazzling it's like moving through fizzy water – cool and clear and luminous. In our back garden, the old plum tree is showing its first blossom. After all it has endured in recent years – having its leaves stripped by possums, having sturdy boughs sawn off by an irritable neighbour who thought the fallen blossom messy – it keeps on giving. Seeing the pale flowers emerge from bare wood never fails to move me. I take photographs, but really it is that determined push of beauty and goodness that I want to remember and emulate.

Extract from my garden journal, August 2021

Chapter 11

Lost in Time

Some years ago, after a family drama left me traumatised, I read that scientists thought they might soon be able to target and erase specific memories. I imagined swallowing something, a 'forgetting pill', while holding in my mind the memory I wanted to erase. Afterwards I would no longer be troubled by the painful scenes from the past. Around the same time as I was wishing to forget events that had caused me such sorrow, an aunt was diagnosed with Alzheimer's. A retired teacher, she changed, with staggering speed, from the capable woman we knew to someone who struggled to remember small but important details, and who after years of being in charge on the domestic front suddenly began to forget how to cook. Her devoted husband cared for her at home, but it was a terrible strain on them both. I remember thinking, after they'd visited me for morning tea, that it was clear you couldn't risk messing with memory and if that meant taking the bad with the good, then so be it.

In Australia nearly one in ten people over sixty-five will suffer dementia. It is sobering to learn that it is the greatest cause of disability in Australians over the age of sixty-five, and among women it is the leading cause of death.

Dementia, with its damaging memory loss, raises our relationship with time, and while much has been written about the way time seems to move slowly when we are young, and speeds up as we grow older, what fascinates me is the way time collapses or becomes fluid in memory. In that mysterious space, fifty years can be bridged in a heartbeat. And if memory is a dimension of time, it is more supple, more forgiving, more maze-like in its turnings and diversions than the relentless forward march measured by clocks.

Clock time propels us towards old age, and death, while the subversive, free-falling element of memory allows us to wander freely in timeless spaces. These are the two kinds of time identified by the French philosopher Henri Bergson, who argued that time has two faces, of which the first, 'objective time', is the time of clocks, calendars and timetables. The second, what Bergson called '*la durée*' ('duration'), is 'subjective time', the time of our inner, lived experience. Crucially, memory holds us in place through both facets of time, which is why the short-term memory loss of Alzheimer's disease is so frightening and disorientating.

But any kind of forgetting is disturbing, and it is not only the ageing mind that accumulates blank stretches. Childhood amnesia is a thing in which, by the age of seven, much of a child's autobiographical experience becomes obscured. A 2013 study carried out by Patricia Bauer and Marina Larkina and published in the *Journal of Experimental Psychology* found that childhood is 'a constant state of forgetting'. This 'accelerated forgetting throughout childhood results in an ever-shrinking pool of memories from early in life', though by the age of eleven the forgetting slows.

It was Sigmund Freud who coined the term 'childhood amnesia', theorising that it was due to repression of traumatic events. What else would we expect from Freud: that was his schtick. Yet childhood amnesia is near universal, surely making it implausible that *everyone* is repressing traumatic memories. Much more likely is the theory of the underdevelopment of the brain structures used for forming and retaining episodic memories, or the incomplete development of language, which facilitates discussion of memories, thus allowing them to become encoded.

As an adult, the forgetting continues, with whole years of my younger life erased of detail. There are standout moments, perhaps reinforced by discussion and repetition, but much of the rest appears lost. These losses make me wish I had kept a journal, and it fuels my commitment to writing one now. Because I can imagine a time when these years will be wiped clean of all the daily events that, while small, have meant so much. Unless I write them down, I will not recall the single chicory flower that appeared on my birthday, or the enormous quince that dropped from the tree onto my upturned face and almost broke my nose. I will forget the cleverness of white cabbage moths seeking camouflage among the quince flowers, and all the rich detail of the seasons.

When pondering ageing and memory, one always returns to our relationship with time, and I can't decide whether I am in sympathy with the inhabitants of the Norwegian island of Sommarøy, where they proposed to abolish it. When one is positioned north of the Arctic Circle, with sixty-nine summer days when the sun does not set, and winters in which it never rises, time as measured by daylight and darkness makes little sense. Visitors have taken to discarding their watches on the bridge that connects the island to the mainland, but human bodies have their own internal cycles: studies show that our organs respond to day and night independently of our brains; they are their own time-keepers. As for Sommarøy, it transpires that the proposal to abolish time on the island was a publicity stunt designed to attract greater numbers of tourists – an appeal to our human desire to wrest back control of time's passage.

In *Women Rowing North*, psychotherapist Mary Pipher reassuringly insists that although we may experience memory deterioration and loss as we grow older, there is a deepening in minds that have 'become less cluttered and more concerned with essentials'. Pipher says: 'Like an old river, our memories run deep and clear. We can see the relationships between things that happened fifty years ago and the ways we react today.' She remarks on a greater ability to make connections.

One thing that seems to soothe those who are afflicted with a deteriorating memory is being in familiar surroundings. As my mother's memory became less than perfect, I saw that she was happiest at home, and it has been the same with another aunt, who at ninety-seven is suffering from much reduced recall. Familiarity as comfort and memory prompt is the guiding premise of *Time Shelter*, the International Booker Prize–winning novel by Bulgarian writer Georgi Gospodinov. In it, a geriatrician builds a 'clinic of the past', decorating each of its floors in a replica of different decades of the 20th century. The familiarity offers Alzheimer's sufferers the chance to feel at home, and the book asks whether our memories of the past can shield us from the chaos of our present.

Working against familiarity is the common practice of moving house after retirement. In some cases it's a downsizing for practical purposes, and may not mean a move away from a known community. But there is the other sort of move, one in which retirees up sticks and take themselves to an entirely different suburb, town or even to a different country.

The downsize and removal to a new location has become one of the clichés of retirement planning, and our lives are so strewn with clichéd thoughts and ideas that it is difficult to steer a way through. To live cliché-free requires confidence and commitment. Take the almost universally accepted belief that it is important to 'get away', or that once we are relieved of the need to go out to work, we will want to travel. But what is it that it is so important for us to get away from? Is it, perhaps, ourselves we seek to escape? Those personas we have partly constructed, and which are partly formed from the constant rub of the niches we inhabit at home? And if home is so terrible that we need to get away, shouldn't we be doing something about that?

In Fiona McFarlane's novel *The Night Guest*, when Ruth's husband Harry announces that on his retirement they should move permanently to their holiday house, the reader registers Ruth's small, involuntary protest: '"Oh no," said Ruth, without thinking. "Really? What would we do all day?"' But her husband goes ahead anyway. 'Harry retired, and they moved, and all day they were Ruth and Harry.'

An outback pastor I once interviewed told me that a big part of his job was counselling 'grey nomad' couples who had sold up and set off around Australia. Often, they are not many months on the road before the cracks appear in their projected retirement happiness. Typically, women mourn the loss of time spent with children and grandchildren. Then, without the conversational outlets of friends and neighbours, couples take to venting with each other. Meanwhile, the cash from the sale of the family home slowly trickles away, raising fears about ever being able to replace it. There must be women who have found themselves on the far side of the continent in a caravan when their husbands unexpectedly die, like Harry in *The Night Guest*. The impulse to get away seems like a sign of self-dissatisfaction dressed up as adventure.

The American journalist and screenwriter Nora Ephron had not reached seventy when she published her final book of essays, *I Remember Nothing*. In the short title piece, Ephron recounts how if she goes to see a play or a film for a second time, 'it's as if I didn't see it at all the first time, even if the first time was just recently'. She laments that 'the past is slipping away' and that her faulty memory makes her feel old. 'I used to think my problem was that my disk was full; now I'm forced to conclude that the opposite is true: it's becoming empty.'

With a flash of dark humour, she remarks that she is living in the 'Google years' and that there are distinct advantages to it: 'When you forget something, you can whip out your iPhone and go to Google. The Senior Moment has become the Google Moment, and it has a much nicer, hipper, younger, more contemporary sound'. Ephron was seventy-one when she died, two years after the book's publication.

In *At Seventy*, May Sarton, an avid gardener, writes of Basil de Sélincourt, the reviewer of her first book of poems, that he taught her 'how to garden into very old age by working at an extremely slow tempo'. For Sarton, very old age was still to come, but she hoped that, like Basil, she would put in a vegetable garden in her late eighties. Gardening, for her, was 'an instrument of grace' and the natural world was the great teacher.

May Sarton was the pen name of the American poet, novelist and memoirist Eleanore Marie Sarton. Born in 1912 in Belgium, she was the only child of the English artist Mabel Eleanor Elwes and the science historian George Sarton. When the Germans invaded Belgium in 1914 the family fled to England, and from there to Boston. By her death in 1995, Sarton had published fifty-three books, and I had never read any of them until I stumbled across her journals.

~

Of all the birds that come into my garden, the blackbird is my favourite. When a female visits the pond garden, I watch her darting between the shrubs and hope that she will bring a mate. I miss the dawn-to-dusk singing, and can't wait to hear it again next spring. 'O'Carolan's Farewell to Music' or blackbird song – it is a toss-up as to which would be my preferred last earthly sound.

I start to think about this in earnest over a cup of tea on the front veranda – the possibility that I might die on an autumn afternoon when there is no blackbird song. I sit there sick with grief and foreboding until I remember that towards the end of spring, when the black songster gave one of his most impassioned performances, I crept up beside the brush fence and recorded him. I didn't do it with dying in mind, but now that I can listen to him sing whenever I want, it has disarmed that particular spectre.

The trouble with dying is that there is no guarantee it won't be messy. I am haunted by the statistic that dementia is the leading cause of death among Australian women, and wonder whether it explains why demented older women occur more frequently in fiction than women ageing well: dementia is a fate that stalks us all, but in books it is rather a stereotype, and I keep hoping to discover novels, and indeed real-life initiatives, that treat dementia differently.

The interim report from the Royal Commission into Aged Care Quality and Safety is not reassuring, finding Australia's failing aged-care industry 'a sad and shocking system that diminishes Australia as a nation' and is in urgent need of reform. The commissioners note that Australia has developed an 'ageist mind-set' and a public discourse that is about 'burden, encumbrance, obligation and whether taxpayers can afford to pay for the dependence of older people'.

Clearly, it is not only dying that humans block, but the acceptance that, in time, any of us may need these care services. As a nation we have developed a defensive barrier against the knowledge that our system of aged care is failing great numbers of vulnerable people.

In *A Long Time Coming: Essays on Old Age*, Melanie Joosten writes:

> Residential-care facilities have become places that nobody wants to end up in, essentially holding pens of last resort, and the very fact that they are roundly despised but never revolutionised can be seen as a way of punishing those who have not played the game properly and remained sufficiently independent.

Perhaps cognisant of what might await them, a growing number of people over sixty-five are ending their own lives in the waiting period before entering aged care. The statistics are sobering.

In the quest for innovative treatments for those afflicted with dementia, I came across Japan's Cafe of Mistaken Orders. This twelve-seat cafe in Sengawa, a suburb in western Tokyo, hires elderly people living with dementia to work an hour-long shift once a month. It would appear to be almost unique as a space in which they can interact with the public while feeling as if they are contributing something useful. Inevitably, moments of confusion arise over orders, but a system of coded colours helps, and volunteers work alongside to make sure the scheme runs smoothly.

Another city taking positive steps to become dementia-friendly is Bruges, a small city in the northwestern part of Belgium. Projects include a choir for dementia patients and their carers, and training for shop-owners to help lost or confused people. They aim to make everyday activities, such as grocery shopping or taking public transport, easier for people with dementia, as well as those who care for them. Importantly, they also seek to reduce barriers to carrying on with life at home by offering greater community support.

In Nottingham in the United Kingdom, in 2018, actress Vicky McClure formed a choir to see whether music could make a measurable difference in the lives of dementia patients. The project was filmed as a BBC1 documentary, in which scientific studies measured singers' emotional and physical responses over a three-month period of regular sessions. The result was Our Dementia Choir, and the outcomes were so positive that the choir continues to meet and sing, including at a festival in front of 24,000 people.

In Australia, dementia cafes tend to be volunteer-run places where patients and carers can go to socialise, but an important element appears to be missing: of giving those living with dementia something useful to do. Still, the use of music is more widespread, and its effectiveness is encouraging. A 2009 study by the University of California, Davis, mapped the brain activity of a group of people while they listened to music and was able to identify the region of the brain where memories of the past link with familiar music and emotion. The area – right behind the forehead – is one of the last parts of the brain to atrophy in Alzheimer's disease, and it is hoped the research will help to develop music-based therapy for sufferers.

At the University of Melbourne's National Music Therapy Research Unit, Professor Felicity Baker studies how music, especially singing and songwriting, can be a way for people living with dementia, and their carers, to deal with the disease's distressing symptoms, such as agitation and depression. Working with small groups on a ten-week songwriting study, Professor Baker found that participants remembered the music they had created – that far from forgetting lyrics they'd worked on, they were able to recall them from week to week. A future study will look at collaborative music therapy, such as choir groups, to see how they might affect cognitive function, depression, neurological symptoms and quality of life.

In Canberra, the Alchemy Chorus welcomes people living with dementia who can take part in singing and performing along with a relative or close friend. A not-for-profit association, they are keen to see Alchemy Chorus choirs established in other parts of Australia, and to foster this they offer consultations with their performance and development manager.

Now that I am well and truly within this awful disease's sightline, I am sometimes surprised by a small inner voice saying, 'Please, I'll settle for something else, but just not *that*.' Even facing up to cancer, frightening as that is, does not terrify me in the same way as the prospect of losing my grasp on memory, on who I am and where I've been. Then, too, after a lifetime of striving after an inner calmness, I am daunted by the agitation that often seems to accompany dementia. I'm not sure how soothed I would be by singing, and my hearing loss would make that tricky.

Over coffee with a friend, whose dementia-affected husband is in residential care, she remarks that it seems to affect everyone a little differently. She says that although her husband's memory is damaged, he still hasn't lost his ability to crack a joke. Apparently, before he became ill he was fond of a joke. 'How dementia manifests,' she says, 'seems to depend on the person you were before you got sick.' Her husband has also been a life-long gardener, and in the care facility his windowsill is crammed with small pots, and even teacups, which he has appropriated for his own use. He fills them with soil, and presses in the cuttings he gathers on walks in the gardens.

'It's amazing,' his wife says, 'the strength of that instinct to connect with the natural world.' Her mother, she says, used to do the same. 'Only Mum would snip cuttings from her care home's artificial indoor plants, and then complain bitterly that they weren't growing.' She adds that many of the women patients at her husband's care home pick flowers in the gardens to decorate their walkers. 'Or if there are no fresh flowers, they'll cut out pictures of them from magazines and stick those on instead.'

Despite the depth of devastation wrought by dementia, it seems our response to beauty – be it in music or the natural world – is embedded even deeper. My friend's husband's persistent gardening habit must be, for him, a stable point in a tilting world. If one day I should be similarly afflicted, I hope my love of gardens will also serve as an anchor. In the meantime, I try to keep the neural pathways in working order with the small daily challenges of Wordle and other puzzles, with reading and writing.

What I've taken from the novels and essays I've read hoping for guidance through this difficult terrain of memory, and its loss, is that our end times are not well served by moving to remote locations, or by distant love, and that old women can be far too brave for their own good. As for the death of memory, as I write this there is news that scientists may be on the verge of a breakthrough in the treatment of dementia. Now what a blessing that would be.

On my morning walk I pass a leafless tree in Westall Street, its bare branches like a pair of hands, twiggy fingers cupped to the wintry sky. It's a seasonal offering-up, and I find the simplicity of its shape so moving.

Less lovely is the creaking-hinge sound of the wattlebirds, their intermittent clacking, to which I wake these mornings. They seem to have chased off the honeyeaters and the blackbirds, though I still hear the occasional thread of song.

That's how life is, I guess, some sweet seasons, some less so. Meanwhile, I fill the water bowls and tend to the tasks, as always, lucky to be here, lucky to have this small green haven, thankful for every single day of breath.

Extract from my garden journal, August 2021

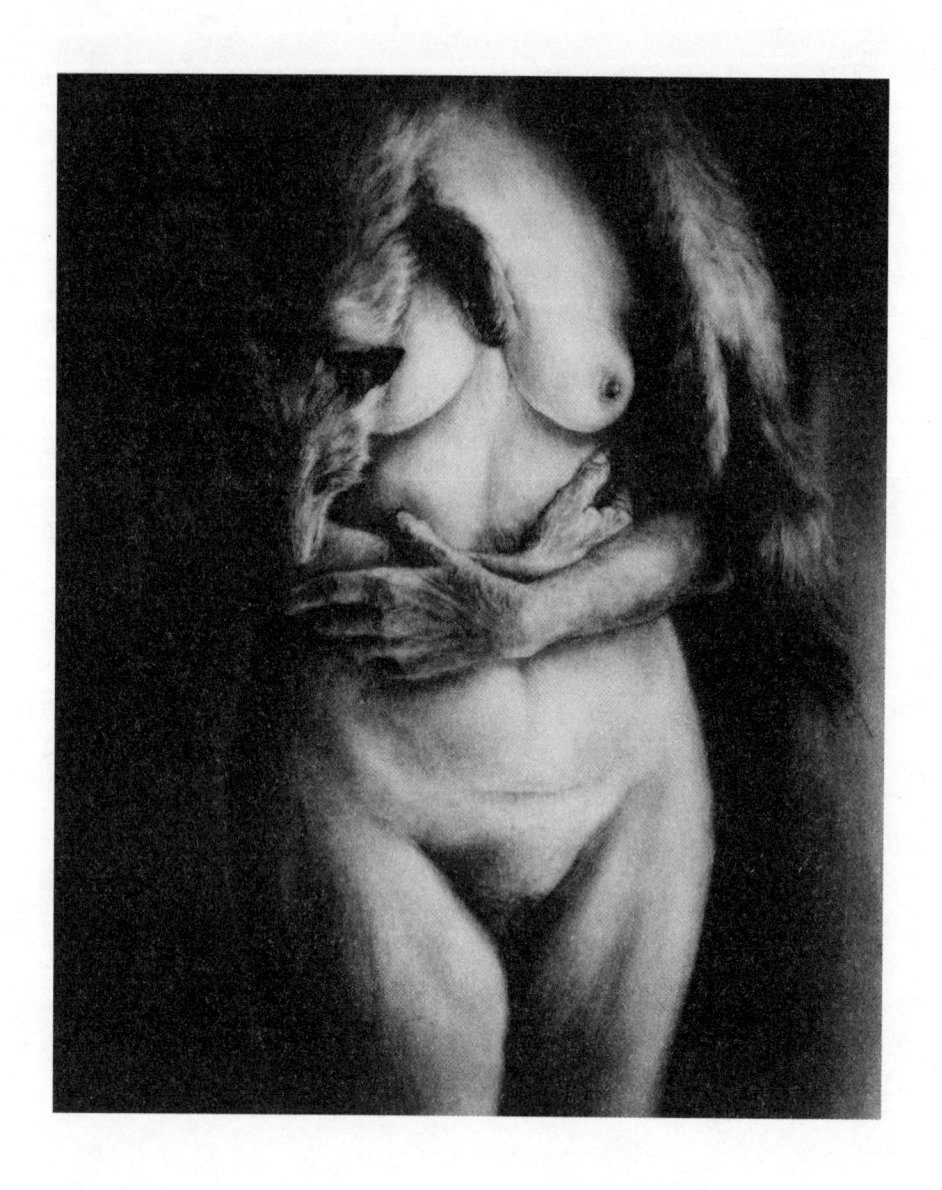

Chapter 12

Love and Age

A friend with a close relative in a residential aged-care home reports – in a tone of scandalised surprise – on romantic entanglements among the elderly. In one case, a man and woman have become so inseparable that staff have been forced to move his bed into her room so the two can sleep side by side. When the woman's son made an unexpected visit, he was distressed to find his mother in her nightdress in the arms of a stranger, though eventually he had to accept it was what she wanted.

The concept of the elderly, with their age-altered bodies, demonstrating an appetite for intimacy, especially in an institutionalised setting, appears widely regarded as funny at best – and at worst disgusting. But should we be surprised if in this difficult, final phase of their lives, elderly people yearn for human contact?

As another friend, an experienced nurse, points out, the rooms of aged-care residents are routinely lined with framed family photographs, what she calls 'the people with the big hats and the scrolls'. But where, my friend demands, are these people in the lives of the lonely residents? Why do they never visit?

She describes how in her childhood in Ireland, any house you'd go to would have an old man or woman in it being cared for by the family; though she admits this may no longer be the case, since so many women have found work outside the home.

For Australians in aged care, living among strangers, removed from all that was once familiar – including the ordinary luxuries of an outing to a local cafe, or to watch the sun set over the sea – it is surely natural that they should turn to those nearest them for comfort.

~

Each February, the Day of Love rolls around, with its buckets of poor, forced roses outside florists, its gaudy greeting cards and supermarkets crammed with chocolate. Young people, of course, are mad for all the hullabaloo, with Valentine's Day parties, and singing telegrams delivered in the lunchbreaks in high schools. But if those young people imagine they have a monopoly on love – or even on sex – the truth appears otherwise, in real life and in books.

Alice Munro's story 'The Bear Came Over the Mountain' is a moving narrative of love at the end of days. It documents both romantic attachment in residential care and the lengths a spouse might go to for love. Grant and Fiona have been married for almost fifty years when she starts leaving sticky notes on their kitchen drawers: *Cutlery, Dishtowels, Knives*. Grant is shaken by the realisation that it is not where things are kept that Fiona is struggling with, but what they are.

As Fiona's memory loss accelerates, she moves voluntarily to Meadowlake, a nursing home where she and Grant have previously visited a neighbour. The home's rules forbid visitors during the first month; Grant is told this is to help Fiona settle in. But when the month is up his wife does not recognise him, and at each visit he finds her sitting close beside her new friend, Aubrey.

Grant's eventual acceptance of Fiona and Aubrey's relationship, and his efforts, after Aubrey's wife takes him home, to have him returned to Meadowlake, is where the real love lies in this story. It is not the stuff of cellophane-wrapped roses and chocolate hearts, but the devotion that accretes over the course of a long marriage. In Grant's case devotion may be tinged with guilt, for in the past he has been a philanderer, though he never wanted to risk losing his wife. Now that he has lost her, he throws his effort into securing the only thing that appears to make her happy.

At the end of Elizabeth Strout's Pulitzer Prize–winning *Olive Kitteridge*, Olive seeks out the widowed Jack Kennison. She puts her hand on his chest and feels the thump of his heart 'and her body – old, big, sagging – felt straight-out desire for his'. Olive is saddened to remember she had not loved her husband Henry in this way for a long time before he died:

> What young people didn't know, she thought, lying down beside this man, his hand on her shoulder, her arm; oh, what young people did not know. They did not know that lumpy, aged, and wrinkled bodies were as needy as their own young, firm ones, that love was not to be tossed away carelessly.

Intimate relationships have been associated with lower levels of stress and depression, with higher levels of oxytocin, a feel-good hormone, and a general lift in physical and mental wellbeing, even taking into account cognitive or physical impairment. Intimacy, of course, does not necessarily mean sex; it can be expressed through touch, such as hugging, cuddling or hand-holding. But in an Australian aged-care setting, this may not be as straightforward as it seems in fiction. For one thing, there is a discouraging lack of privacy, including a scarcity of shared rooms, rooms with double beds and lockable doors. Then, if a resident's husband or wife is still living in the wider community, a new attachment will likely stir family resistance.

A recent survey of almost 3000 Australian residential aged-care facilities conducted by researchers at La Trobe University's Australian Centre for Evidence Based Aged Care found that only half of facilities surveyed had written policies on sexuality, and only one-third had policies on sexual behaviour.

Dementia raises the question of a capacity to properly consent. Legislation is clear concerning a resident's will and medical and financial matters. But when it comes to people's sexual decisions, it is left to staff to negotiate a balance between the rights of individuals and the facility's duty of care to a group of people who are particularly vulnerable to unwanted attentions, or even sexual assault.

It must be acknowledged that in Australia an estimated fifty sexual assaults occur every week in residential aged care, and that the elderly also experience such assaults in their own homes; victims are invariably female. Police and care providers can be unwilling to act, believing that dementia makes the victim's evidence unreliable – and, mistakenly, that people with dementia will not remember, nor be traumatised.

The Ready to Listen project, launched in 2021 by the Older Persons Advocacy Network, aims to address the rights of people in aged care to be heard, to be believed, and (following open disclosure of assault) to have their cases followed up by police. It is also concerned with establishing a charter of sexual rights for older people, including their right to a consensual, romantic relationship, and clarifying the all-important question of consent.

But the possibility of non-consensual contact exacerbates the difficulty of forming genuine attachments, and family disapproval may be enough to cause staff to intervene. Even without this, the lack of guidance, or the ageist prejudices of staff members, may mean intimate friendships within an aged care setting will be firmly discouraged.

Children, especially adult children, can complicate mature love, and are often unscrupulous in thwarting it. Because aside from what they perceive as age-inappropriate behaviour, late-life attachments can, of course, have consequences for an offspring's anticipated inheritance.

In Kent Haruf's *Our Souls at Night*, Addie Moore and Louis Waters, neighbours for years, both live alone: their houses empty of family, their evenings solitary. Then Addie visits Louis with the astonishing proposal that he sleep over with her at night – for the company, for the quiet conversations after lights out. Louis agrees, and they fall into a companionable routine. The town soon notices this new intimacy but, at seventy, Addie does not care what anyone thinks, nor does Louis.

Alerted by a friend to her father's behaviour, Louis's daughter Holly tells him, "'It just seems embarrassing.'" But Addie's son Gene takes a darker view of the relationship. He confronts his mother: "'If you married him he'd get half of everything, wouldn't he? I couldn't stop him.'"

Addie's six-year-old grandson Jamie is sent to stay with her when Gene separates from his wife. Frightened at night, Jamie ends up sleeping in Addie's bed, making her arrangement with Louis impossible. But gradually the three of them bond, and when Louis gives Jamie a dog, Bonny, Bonny is allowed to sleep on Jamie's bed. When the three of them go camping, they share the same tent.

Gene comes and takes Jamie and Bonny. "'I want this to stop,' he says. "You're not even ashamed of yourselves.'" He bans Addie from speaking on the phone to her grandson. When she does get through to Jamie, he tells her that if he talks to her, 'they'll take Bonny away'. Addie must have contact with the boy; she cannot afford to wait until Jamie is sixteen. She tells Louis they must remain separate.

When Addie falls in the street, Gene has her transferred from the town of Holt, where she and Louis live, to Denver. Louis goes to the hospital, where Gene tells him, "'You're not wanted here.'" When Addie is discharged, she will move into assisted living in another town. Gene's disgust, while partly motivated by financial need, is also an expression of a common distaste for age-altered bodies. To Gene, this is all the justification he needs to use his small son as a weapon.

Addie Moore is not the first elderly woman to discover that the last great love of her life is a grandchild. The unconditional love can flow both ways, to mutual joy, if it is not pinched out by parents with a loveless attitude towards the older generation. In her surrealist novel *The Hearing Trumpet*, Leonora Carrington delivers this dehumanising impulse with devastating economy as a woman speaks to her husband about his aged mother, Marian.

"'Remember, Galahad,' added Muriel, "those old people do not have feelings like you or I. She would be so much happier in an institution."'

Unfortunately for Marian, her adult grandson is not the loving kind. '"She ought to be dead," Robert said. "At that age people are better off dead."'

Even when offspring are not primarily focused on their inheritance, there can be a lifetime's accumulation of feelings and resentments in play. In *Anything Is Possible*, also by Elizabeth Strout, in the story 'Mississippi Mary', a seventy-eight-year-old woman lives in Italy, married to a man so much younger than her that at first the locals assume she is his mother.

When her youngest daughter visits, Mary thinks she will not understand 'what it had been like to be so famished. Almost fifty years of being parched.' At their fiftieth wedding anniversary party her husband had not asked her to dance. Later, when Mary was sixty-nine, her daughters had given her a trip to Italy as a birthday gift, and it was there that she had wandered off and become lost, and was found by Paolo.

'She fell in love. She did. He'd been married for twenty years, it had seemed like fifty to him, and now he was alone – they were both parched.'

Mary's first husband had been in a long-term affair. Their daughter Angelina judges it 'pathetic ... painful, of course, but pathetic'. Her father, Angelina admits, 'really was a mean snake of a man' but then the selfishness of the hurt child kicks in: 'Why couldn't her mother see what she had done by leaving? Why couldn't she see it?'

Angelina accuses her mother of having taken from her the ability to care for her in her old age, and to be with her when she dies. Mary is a little stricken by this, because she suspects death is not far away. But 'she did not dread her death ... she was almost ready for it, not really but getting there'. She admits that 'Always, there was that grasping for a few more years, Mary had seen this with many people, and she did not feel it – or she did, but she did not. No. She felt tired out, she felt almost ready, and she could not tell her child this.'

May Sarton famously developed the optimistic concept of 'ripening towards death in a fruitful way'. But ripeness as it relates to the elderly, especially elderly women, can be a fraught topic. Some pro-ageing advocates insist that an essential element of a woman ageing well is glamour, but glamour is a construct; in our times it is often measured by the subject's perceived sexual appeal.

The pro-ageing movement on Instagram is divided between older women who still prefer the familiar accessories of their youth – skin-baring garments, high heels, makeup – and those who are evolving towards a kind of beauty that focuses instead on being comfortable in one's own skin. Neither approach is right or wrong, but of the two ways of going forward, the less-is-more philosophy of the natural agers somehow seems more universally doable.

The roots of the word 'glamour' can be traced to the Scottish word *gramarye*, meaning 'magic, enchantment, spell', including the lovely phrase 'to cast the glamour'. *Gramarye* may be from an Ancient Greek word for the weight unit of ingredients used in magic potions. Or it may be an alteration of the English word 'grammar', in its medieval sense of 'scholarship' and especially 'occult learning'.

In John Jamieson's *Etymological Dictionary of the Scottish Language*, from 1825, glamer, glamour, is 'the supposed influence of a charm on the eye, causing it to see objects differently from what they really are. Hence to 'cast glamer o'er one, to cause deception of sight'. This definition draws glamour closer to the Old Norse words *glámr* – 'moon' or 'name of a ghost' – and *glámsýni* – 'illusion' – which makes of glamour a deception, a beauty trick.

Jamieson's dictionary contains many old words that women might use to describe themselves, in ways that stand outside the conventions formed around youthful beauty. For those of us anticipating our own extreme old age, when we will be more *frooch* ('frail, brittle') than now, let us hope we shall still be able to summon the odd moment of *gleit* ('to glitter'), and that our eyes, our hair, will be touched at times with their old *glister* ('lustre'). Looking back over the fiction I've drawn on for this chapter, I see the writers were both *forsy* ('powerful') and *formois* ('beautiful').

~

In March 1986, in the Euroa Hostel in northern Victoria, First World War veteran Jim Sinclair, eight-nine, and Lily Schoon, eighty-eight, were banned by the Shire Council from meeting in their rooms, or even eating together. The couple, who had met at the hostel four years earlier, insisted that they were just good friends. At the time, Lily, a great-grandmother, was partially blind and walked with the aid of a stick.

'I think the world of him,' she said. 'Without Jim, I don't know where I'd be.'

Among rules put in place by the council were 'Rule 14: Any social visiting between residents is to be encouraged in the lounges only. Rule 15: Visitors are permitted entry to bedrooms only because of ill health of the resident, or the approval of the supervisor. Door to remain open during visit.'

Lily had been used to going to Jim's room every day to watch TV, but the hostel supervisor, Mrs Sibson, banned the visits.

'We're not running a brothel,' she said. 'I'm not going to allow it to get to that stage.'

A Health Commission spokesman, when told of the rules, said, 'It doesn't look like a happy home-like atmosphere, does it?'

When asked for comment, Jim, who had been a prisoner of war, shook his head. 'I reckon the Germans treated me better than this lot.'

The Royal Commission into Aged Care Quality and Safety was announced in 2018, following a string of disturbing incidents – including South Australia's Oakden Aged Care scandal, after which the facility was closed when evidence came to light of neglect and abuse. Among the findings of the Royal Commission was that 'sub-standard care and abuse pervades the Australian aged care system'. In its final report, it pronounced this 'a source of national shame'. Reforms suggested by the Royal Commission in any overhaul of Australia's aged-care system include the right of autonomy, the right to the presumption of legal capacity, and in particular the right of elders in residential aged care to make decisions about their care and the quality of their lives, and the right to social participation.

The recommendations state that older people should be supported to exercise choice about their own lives and make decisions to the fullest extent possible, including being able to take risks and be involved in the planning and delivery of their care. They also state that older people are entitled to receive support that acknowledges the aged-care setting is their home, and enables them to live in security, safety and comfort, with their privacy respected.

For those of us who are not yet ready to access these late-life services, let us hope the current government follows through on the Royal Commission's recommendations, which declare that people should be treated as individuals. And that the relationships older people have with significant others in their lives should be acknowledged, fostered and respected.

The garden is in the grip of winter, yet there is a faint hum of anticipation; it is like a theatre at intermission. In the mornings, light pours in and fills the space between the trees and the house and the brush fence. It is too cold to sit out on the veranda, but I watch from my study window.

This is the time to rest and to dream; it is also the time to travel to other gardens, to wallow deep and long in the writings of other gardeners.

Extract from my garden journal, August 2021

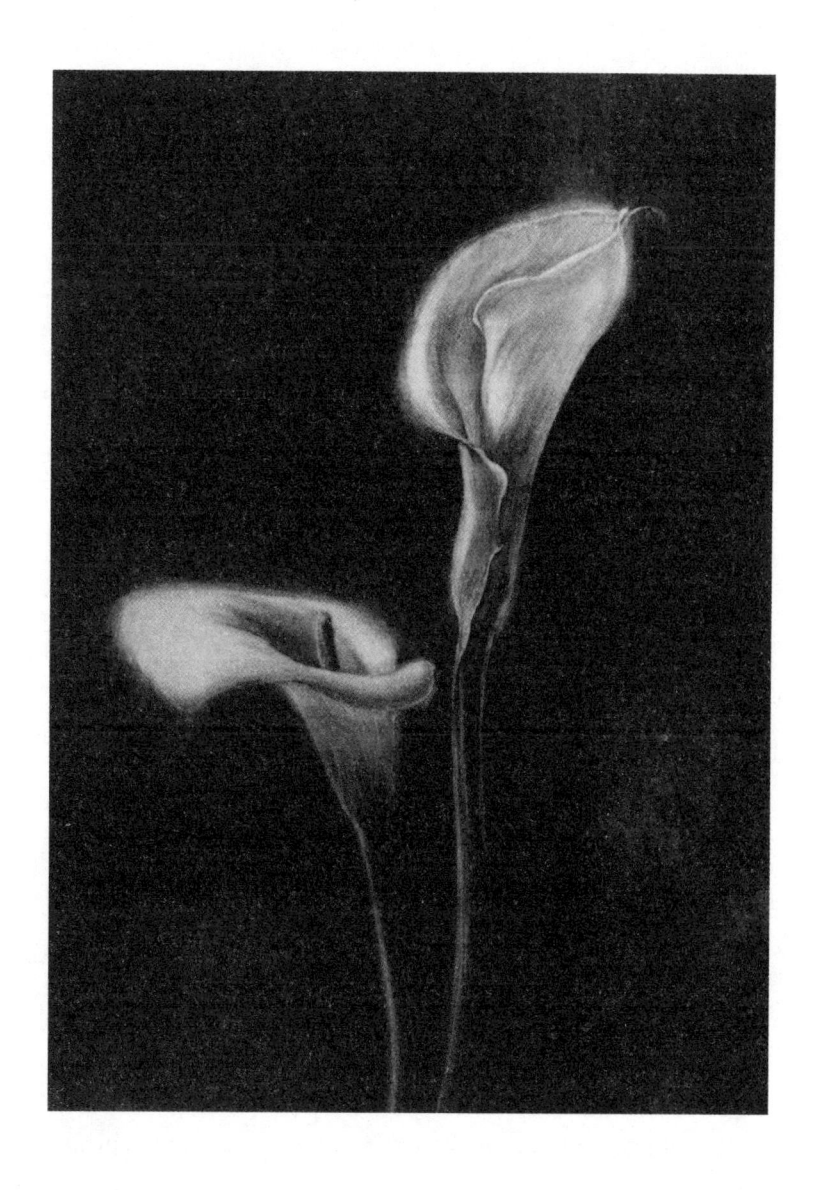

Chapter 13

The View from the Tower

Age and loneliness

For an old woman in the forty-third year of her marriage, the possibility of one day having to live alone is like trying to visualise making a new life for myself on the moon. It fills me with dread, and I wonder about my resilience. The truth is, I don't know how I will cope with late-life grief and loneliness, if that should be the card I'm dealt.

The Japanese writer Haruki Murakami has said, 'In a sense our lives are nothing more than a series of stages to help us get used to loneliness.' Daunting as this idea may be, many of us will face varying states of loneliness as we age, so it would make sense to prepare for it. But can such a thing as loneliness ever be prepared for? My first thought is that it can't, but then commonsense whispers that the thing I dread is not a random, unforeseeable event. It is the outcome of time's ruthlessness, which threatens to deprive me, one by one, of the people I hold dear.

Like most everyone, I've spent a lifetime attempting to deny or ignore this threat, whistling and looking the other way, perfecting my terror management.

When I do allow the dread to surface, it often takes the form of a mental image of a tarot card: the Tower. A tower struck by lightning, with flames leaping in its windows, while two doomed figures plunge towards the ground. The Tower has a reputation as the most feared card in the tarot deck, worse even than the image of that skeletal grim reaper, Death. Because the Death card, in its benign aspects, can simply signify a change of horses, the ending of one thing and the beginning of another, whereas the Tower represents unforeseen catastrophe, ways of living not just changing but being violently demolished.

Whether or not you believe in the tarot deck as a predictive tool – and I view it in much the same way as astrology: interesting, but impossible to prove – its charm lies in the iconography of its images and symbols, which represent forces, characters, virtues and vices, as they relate to aspects of the human condition. Each card is a mini masterpiece of design that cleverly taps into our deepest fears and desires and sets them neatly before us on a playing card. For me, the Tower is as graphic a depiction as I can summon of the dread with which I contemplate significant late-life change and loss, and the resulting loneliness.

~

I watched my mother's gradual ascent towards loneliness. It kicked in early for her, when at forty-seven she was widowed. Her mother died not long after, followed some years later by her father. Her beloved older sister went next, which was, perhaps, the hardest parting of all, as they had been extraordinarily close since childhood. Her younger brother's death left my mother – the middle child – as the last of her immediate family. There had been, as well, the falling-away of those friends who had once dropped in for tea and cake and chats, or who came to the candlelit dinner parties she loved to throw, even though she insisted she was not much of a cook. Once the setting for convivial gatherings, through her eighties and nineties my mother's old house gradually fell silent.

In childhood games of this nature there would be a prize for the survivor, but for those who reach an extreme old age, having lost parents, siblings and contemporaries who knew them when they were young, even the presence of children and grandchildren may not erase their last-man-standing loneliness. My mother carried herself throughout with dignity; she was reticent in her grief. But she'd often say that four days at home alone was about her limit. I like to think we never allowed her to reach the four-day mark.

During what proved to be the last decade of her life I began to think of my mother as a lonely queen in a lonely tower. It was an image prompted in part by her composure, the small white head that looked as if it would continue to bear up, even under the weight of a jewel-encrusted, golden crown. A sense of remoteness clung to her like an invisible cloak, so that although we were together it was as if those hours she spent alone never entirely dissipated. She might have been looking out at a far landscape, one we could not catch a glimpse of from our different vantage points.

By ninety-five she had begun a subtle withdrawal, turning down the volume on life and retreating more and more into a private world that perhaps was populated by her lost loved ones. Still living independently, for the most part she seemed untouched by cognitive decline, yet she deflected or dismissed my questions about the past, always insisting she couldn't remember. I thought she was being evasive, that she saw the past as painful. But now I wonder whether there was a decline in memory that I'd failed to notice, or had not wanted to notice.

I began to think and write about towers around that time, and about the women who might inhabit them. Because statistics show that women, with their longer lifespans, are generally left to inhabit the sparsely populated spaces at life's last knockings. *The Tower* is the first book of mine that my mother will never read. In it, an elderly widow, Dorelia, finds that the house she shared with her husband during a long marriage has become distressing to her in his absence. Every mirror holds fragments of him, and she'd like to cover all of them with cloths if not for her adult children, who might think she isn't holding up. Instead, against their wishes, Dorelia sells the family home and moves into an unsuitable house with a tower. Driving my writing was a desire to give to this fictional character something I was helpless to give my mother – a place where all the grief she had been carrying simply fell away, and she could abide in peace and calm.

Years earlier, I had photographed a round tower at Killala in the west of Ireland, a structure in which, at the first sign of attack, the whole town had been able to shelter. It had lodged in my consciousness as a symbol of refuge, a place to flee to in times of strife. Yet gradually, its iconic shape has merged in my thinking with other tower-like structures we inhabit throughout our lives – childhood, family, friendship, marriage, memory, the past, old age and that loneliest of fortresses: the stronghold of the self.

My mother's widowhood, and even the fictional Dorelia's, prompt me to wrestle with my dread. I think back to the time when I found myself living in an unfamiliar city, far from everyone I knew. I had bolted after the breakdown of a youthful and doomed relationship, and the state of darkness I fell into through one desolate stretch over the New Year, and my birthday, remains vivid. To face a similar season as an old woman would test my resilience, perhaps even to breaking point.

The experience of that loneliness sits in my memory like a black-and-white still from an old film. I remember the small round table in the kitchen of my flat, where I sat hugging my guitar and drinking endless cups of instant coffee. But it was when I first began to write, and the entire adventure marked the beginning of my independent life: free of the influence of my family's thoughts and ideas about how I should live; free, even, of the culture I had been raised in. The price I paid for striking out on my own was that for a long time 'home' became an ill-defined and shifting concept, a mirage, longed for yet understood to be not a matter of simply 'going back': home, I sensed, would have to be rebuilt somehow, from materials and resources I did not yet possess.

The emotion of loneliness was immobilising, but I see now that instead of moping in the kitchen I should have gone for a few good long walks in the botanic gardens across the road. Perhaps this sterner view, the certainty that exercise has the power to shift difficult emotions through and out of our bodies, shows that my resilience has increased over the intervening decades.

~

Loneliness is felt as a profound and painful yearning for connection. In her book *The Lonely City*, Olivia Laing describes it as 'like being hungry when everyone around you is readying for a feast. It feels shameful and alarming, and over time these feelings radiate outwards, making the lonely person increasingly isolated.' Laing talks about the shame of loneliness, describing it as 'a taboo state that will cause others to turn and flee'. People who are lonely often try to keep it a secret; they fear appearing weird or needy. This can lead them to become hypervigilant for signs of rejection, which in turn leads to rejecting behaviours. In this way, loneliness forms a persistent cycle.

A research paper by the pioneering German psychiatrist Frieda Fromm-Reichmann refers to the process of 'incorporation and identification', used to counteract the loneliness following a bereavement. In this defensive behaviour, a person mourning the loss of a loved one comes to develop a likeness 'in looks, personality, and activities' to the lost beloved. In this way they fight their loneliness.

I read this with a ping of recognition, remembering how after my mother's death I clung to the things that had belonged to her. On most days, I carried with me one of the soft cotton handkerchiefs she favoured. I wore her hand-knitted jumpers, spritzed her perfume. I found comfort in the steady tick of her wristwatch and bedside clock, and the fact I was so often told how much I look like her.

~

Not so long ago, it was common for old people to be cared for at home, absorbed into a son's or a daughter's household. The granny flat was a ubiquitous addition to suburban houses. Historically, it had evolved from the Victorian dower house, a separate dwelling on an estate where the owner's widow could remain on familiar soil after his death, while ownership of the main house passed to the new heir.

Much less grand than the dower house, the granny flat's purpose was to accommodate an elderly relative who was no longer able to live alone but not yet ready to enter a nursing home. But with the rise of the aged-care industry, and the changing nature and makeup of families, the granny flat began to fall out of favour. Small self-contained dwellings at the bottom of our suburban gardens, spaces that might once have housed an ageing parent, are now more likely to function as studios, or home offices.

If we, or our old people, are lonely, surely it is an outcome of the way we live in the first quarter of the 21st century: more tuned to the 'self' than to the family group (if there is a functioning group). Family networks stretch nationwide, or even globally. But families themselves break down, or become so complex in their connections and loyalties that they often cannot provide a safety net for those members who encounter serial losses and find themselves alone.

But our loneliness is quietly driving change. In Australia, co-housing schemes are creating intentional communities. This means living either in a collection of private homes, accompanied by communally owned shared spaces, or in developments of self-contained dwellings, arranged within common areas for shared activities. Communal living, or co-housing, is a revival of the village model that arguably served our ancestors better than our current individualism is serving us. As we push deeper into the century, and our population ages, co-housing, or versions of it, is likely to become a mainstream housing form, and a viable solution for those for whom old age might otherwise be a lonely place.

Meanwhile, in anticipation of a future shortage of aged-care housing, the federal government has encouraged both state and local governments to simplify the planning regulations for the construction of granny flats.

~

What measures can we take to shore up our lives against future loneliness? Is forewarned forearmed? By looking ahead and accepting the possibility that loneliness might come knocking, we could work harder at building new friendships. We could introduce more sociability into our lives before we even really need it: by volunteering, or embracing a group activity such as a walking club or a choir, or by taking a class.

Recently, delivering a bundle of bedding to Vinnies, I was directed to a receiving area, where all the people in sight within the cavernous warehouse were elderly. A small army of them was receiving and sorting donations. In another part of the building, other elderly volunteers were selling clothing and bric-a-brac. It is the same when I visit the Oxfam second-hand bookshop. Voluntary labour largely goes unnoticed, but without it most charities couldn't function. By joining in and doing good for others, we could also be doing good for ourselves.

It helps, too, to remember that there are people all around us who doubtless feel the same. We never know what is going on in the background of the lives we brush up against. A greeting and a smile could go a long way towards making someone feel that the world is not an entirely hostile place.

I've managed my own lonely times by reading. A good book offers a world one can sink into and become part of. Books – and public libraries

– can be places for the lonely to shelter. But reading is a solitary pastime, and to treat loneliness through reading one would ideally join a book club or discussion group, so the activity can be shared. Perhaps the surest antidote is to develop, if not a love of being alone, then at least a tolerance for it, and find ways to make our alone time fruitful. As we age, we'd be wise to cling fiercely to the skills acquired over a lifetime and continue to develop them. We should also consider taking up new ones.

With typical melancholy and pragmatism, Murakami insists: 'The older a person gets, the lonelier he becomes. It's true for everyone. That being the case, there's no reason to complain. And besides, who would we complain to, anyway?'

Only ourselves, I suppose. But recent statistics appear not to support Murakami's assertion, with surveys – perhaps surprisingly – finding that people over sixty-five are the least lonely. Of course, there exists the possibility that the statistics are skewed by generational differences, that older people are just more stoic, more habituated to their solitude and less comfortable revealing loneliness, even in an anonymous survey.

I ask myself as I write this: am I ever lonely? The answer is sometimes. Because writing is a solitary practice. It takes me out of the world for hours and days at a stretch. I write in a house I live in with two other people, whom I can go to at any time for company and conversation. But the stark reality that shadows our small household's happiness is that one day I will lose them, or they will lose me. What is to become of the one of us who remains?

With this question, my dread kicks in again. But lately, instead of pressing it down, or turning to some form of terror management, I've tried speaking back to it with lines from a poem by Rainer Maria Rilke:

'Let everything happen to you: beauty and terror. / Just keep going. No feeling is / final.'

To just keep going is such simple yet profound advice. And at seventy I know that no feeling, however extreme, ever *is* final. Everything passes and, if you keep on breathing, resilience kicks in.

Beyond resilience is the concept of antifragility. While 'resilient' relates to something or someone robust enough to withstand shock or disruption, 'antifragile' describes a state beyond resilience, in which a thing improves or becomes stronger when harmed. In *Antifragile: Things that Gain from Disorder*, Nassim Nicholas Taleb explains antifragility with the example of human muscles, or bones, that become stronger when subjected to the stress of lifting or bearing weights. To become antifragile in old age could serve us well.

The sorrows that have come my way have been uncomfortable, but in weathering them I've become stronger. Without the chaos and catastrophe, with nothing to push back against, I'd still be some version of that gormless girl strumming sad songs on her guitar.

In the garden, pruning is an antifragile activity. In the early lives of my fruit trees, it often appeared brutal, and yet look how robust they've grown, how they are laden with fruit. The roses, too, respond to the tough love of the pruning shears. I often marvel at the miraculous nature of seeds. Withered flowers reducing to seedheads that look all but dead, yet which contain all the genetic material to birth new flowers. Even when picked and stored, seeds can lie dormant for years and still germinate to fill a garden.

My mother's early widowhood was a form of chaos and disruption she would rather have done without. Yet after a time, following the deaths of both her parents, she returned as a mature student to art school. It was a dream she'd been denied in girlhood, when she was sent to business college to learn shorthand and typing like so many other young women of her generation. Her joy in drawing and painting, and in the photography as fine art that eventually became her major subject at graduation, was an antifragile response to the earlier harm.

In time, if I or one of my dear ones should draw the Tower card, with its fiery image of lives dismantled, implicit in it will be the rebuild that must follow destruction and demolition – antifragility rather than mere resilience. Somehow, within each of us, the materials to rebuild must be found. Because whatever happens in this one extraordinary life we have been given, it is necessary to just keep going, to fully inhabit it to the end.

Go outside and dig a little hole, and put these hurts into it with the clary sage that needs to be planted out.

Extract from my garden journal, August 2021

Chapter 14

Finding Shelter

In writing about what my garden means to me I am acutely aware that even in a country with so much apparent space as Australia, a garden of one's own is not available to everyone. Nor does everyone have the luxury of permanent shelter. I try to imagine what it would have felt like to be discharged from hospital after surgery with nowhere private to retreat to. No couch in front of the fire, no kitchen to make nourishing meals, no warm bed to crawl into at the end of each day, or whenever the world felt overwhelming. And if I lived alone there would have been no one to ask whether I'd like a cup of tea, or to just sit quietly with me through the healing process.

Loneliness is one thing, but homelessness quite another. I'd like to say that my life has never been touched by it, but that would not be true. As a young woman I often lived precariously, setting off with misguided bravado to far-flung places, mostly with precious few resources. I may have been convinced of my own invincibility, but if I didn't find employment soon after arrival, I was in trouble. I remember my shock and dismay after a week in a new job in New Zealand, on discovering that I was to be paid fortnightly. I was a full week away from being able to buy groceries, and during that testing second week I would rise early in the mornings and make the long walk to work to save the bus fare, passing cafes and bakeries whose scent of the freshly baked bread I could not afford set my stomach rumbling. A few years later, on an ill-judged trip to South Africa, I was only saved from certain starvation by a chance encounter with another traveller from whom I learned of a seasonal vacancy, a live-in job in a coastal hotel. Over those years there were many hand-to-mouth days in which I was often stressed about accommodation, but I was never reduced to sleeping in my car, or in a public park.

In Australia, on any given night, around 122,494 people are homeless, and when we think of those affected what springs to mind is an image of figures camped in doorways, or in parks. But to be homeless does not necessarily mean one is 'roofless', and the majority of homelessness is hidden, with people living in crisis accommodation or rooming houses or couch surfing. For women, it is often domestic violence that propels them into supported accommodation.

In the 2021 census in Australia, one in seven people experiencing homelessness was aged fifty-five and over. Of women fifty-five and over, 27 per cent were staying temporarily in other households and 31 per cent were living in overcrowded dwellings; 8 per cent were sleeping outside. Older men were more often living in boarding houses – 37 per cent – while 12 per cent were in improvised accommodation, such as tents, or sleeping rough.

When we think about how someone might be forced into homelessness, it is often family violence, lives ravaged by drugs and alcohol, or mental health conditions that spring to mind. Darlene O'Leary, a team leader in the mental health programs at a homelessness service for women, explains that older women's homelessness can often be traced back to sexual and other forms of childhood abuse.

'Childhood trauma leads to a lack of a sense of self-worth in adulthood,' Darlene says. 'It predisposes women to enter into relationships in which they are not respected, and in which they become victims of control and coercion, and eventually violence.'

If you're an older woman not directly affected by any of these things, you might imagine you are safe; older working women do not immediately present as at risk of homelessness, yet increasingly – with the scarcity of affordable rental accommodation – they are adding to the numbers. Their decline in fortunes arises from an accumulation of factors over time, which may then be tipped over the edge by some unforeseen life crisis. The scary thing is that homelessness could happen to almost any of us, given the right constellation of misfortunes.

On the list of contributing factors to older women's homelessness is a lifetime of lower earnings, and the gender gap in retirement savings and retirement incomes. Women's choices about paid work have often been limited by childcare concerns, or other caring responsibilities, and many will have found themselves part of the 'sandwich generation', caring for both children and other family members. A survey of 9500 women by the Community and Public Sector Union found that a third of women aged forty-five to sixty-four had 'significant caring responsibility of others – usually their partner, adult children, or parents'.

Moving in and out of the workforce, earning less than men, vulnerable to violence, to sexual harassment in the workplace and to age discrimination, older women need only a major setback – such as the breakdown of a marriage, job loss, the death of a partner or a diagnosis of serious illness – for a pathway to open into homelessness.

It is sobering to realise that when the Australian Human Rights Commission discusses the impact of age discrimination on older women, they are referring to women aged forty-five and over. Discrimination is fed by stereotypes and assumptions about older women workers, including that they 'lack potential, are low in energy, have poor skills, and are socially remote from other staff', so that women in the forty-five to fifty-four age group have 'significantly higher rates of under-utilisation in the paid workforce, compared to their male counterparts'.

Separation and divorce have serious implications for women's housing security, with women's disposable income commonly decreasing following a split. This limits their capacity to accumulate superannuation, or make voluntary savings. Even receiving two-thirds of a couple's assets at divorce does not guarantee women long-term housing security, because of their subsequent inability to meet housing costs. As women living alone in their fifties and sixties, they become vulnerable to any crisis that puts their job at risk. Sometimes it's a health setback, or age discrimination leading to the loss of work. In 2022 the Salvation Army's homelessness services assisted 37,000 people, of which nearly one in twenty were women aged fifty-five and over, the fastest growing cohort among the homeless.

Catherine House, in Adelaide, provides much-needed care and accommodation for women experiencing homelessness. Women who find their way into their programs are met with non-judgemental support, and for many it may be the first time in their lives that they are listened to and treated with respect. The women in their recovery program may have been referred by the courts, by hospitals or other agencies; some will have referred themselves. A small number go on to be permanently supported in communal living situations, but the majority will eventually find a place in social housing, although currently there is a years-long waiting list. Catherine House is unique among such services in that there is no time limit on clients' participation in their programs.

Both loneliness and homelessness are unwelcome outcomes of the way we live now, with family connections stretched and complex. I sense that in our Western society we are more self-focused in this century than in the one that came before, and what this means for old people is that finding a home with one of their children when age makes life difficult may be less likely than it was for earlier generations. As I write this, it feels instinctively 'true', yet when I seek studies to support this opinion I find roughly as many that challenge it as those that agree.

From lived experience I can only offer the fact that none of my grandparents entered aged care; they lived at home until their deaths, cared for by one or more of their children. In Broken Hill, my maternal grandmother nursed her husband's parents in a very small house with few facilities while raising four kids. One of those, my aunt, was seven at the time, and remembers that her mother was pregnant again while caring for the old people, that she gave birth prematurely and that the baby soon died. The labour of aged-care she describes was gruelling, outside help non-existent, conditions so primitive that even when I arrived in that household a dozen or so years later there was only a rickety outdoor dunny to serve the whole family, and my grandmother still cooked on a wood-burning stove.

'You know the way old people poop themselves,' says my aunt. 'Well, Mum would burn sugar in the bedroom to get rid of the smell. She would bring in a shovelful of hot coals and sprinkle the sugar on them – the smell was awful, but the poop was worse.'

Her father had sisters, my aunt recalls, but adds that none of them would take the old people. So it seems there have always been those willing to put what they perceive as duty before self-interest, as well as those determined to put themselves first. Perhaps home care was a working-class ideology. More likely, it was at least partly financial. What I do know is that life was threadbare in those war and post-war years, and I can't imagine where the money would have come from to fund outside residential care, even if it had been available.

If our old age plays out without the live-in support of offspring – and I'm referring to the ageing of my generation of Baby Boomers (people born between 1946 and 1964 whose children are either Generation X or Y (Millennials) depending on when they had them) – perhaps we only have ourselves to blame. Not unfairly, we have been dubbed the 'Me' generation in response to our push for individualism as we grew to adulthood amid the social upheaval of the sixties and what Tom Wolfe has described in *New York Magazine* as 'the Me Decade' of the seventies. Perhaps inevitably, those who toyed with 'self-realisation' and 'finding' themselves in those hedonistic decades went on to raise children who would take the push for individualism even further: Millennials, according to *Time* magazine, are the 'Me Me Me Generation'.

Unflatteringly portrayed as having been raised to believe that they were special – famously presented with medals for taking part rather than for winning – Millennials are noted for prioritising individual 'life choices'; some psychologists, such as Jean Twenge, author of *Generation Me*, have flagged an inflated sense of entitlement and the rise of narcissism.

Despite these criticisms, many Boomer offspring – whether Gen X-ers, the micro-generation known as Xennials or the more numerous Millennials – are already stepping up to care for ageing parents. Go to Google and you'll find reports of adult children moving back into the parental home as the most economically viable solution to providing aged care. Heartbreakingly, you'll also come across forums where family breakdown, estrangement and bitter feuds fuel the view that no care is owed, or will be given.

If this latter seems sad and harsh, a balancing article in the journal of the Gerontological Society of America, 'Millennials and Their Parents: Implications of the New Young Adulthood for Midlife Adults', considers the changes in the nature of young adulthood that will impact on parents' future ageing. It finds that grown offspring are staying at home longer; they're marrying later and delaying having children. What this seems to mean is a stronger bond between parent and child, with the possibility that an increased intimacy will evolve into a willingness to provide late-life care.

On the other hand the article notes that 'parents may be less able to obtain such care due to demographic changes involving grown children raising their own children later or who have never fully launched'. In the end it seems impossible to say for sure that any one outcome is 'true' of current social trends. Outcomes will be many and varied, as loving or as bitter as the relationships – practical, emotional and financial – that underpin families.

Community living looks like a viable alternative to moving in with family, especially for older single women. It's not a new concept, and has a precedent in the Beguines of medieval Europe – Roman Catholic women who devoted themselves to prayer and good works, but without taking vows. By forming small collectives, unmarried older women, usually widows, avoided living in poverty, or entering the convent as a nun.

In our own century, in the United States, the Golden Girls Network was a database of single older adults, both women and men, willing to home-share with compatible others. The founder of the network, Bonnie Moore, came up with the idea after renovating her home, only for her marriage to break down. Left with a mortgage she could not afford just as the 2008 global financial crisis hit, she started looking for roommates, and eventually found herself in business helping others to start their own Golden Girls Homes.

Share houses were a common feature of life in the seventies, so their re-emergence is a return to a way of living many of us were once familiar with and might cheerfully embrace again. Moore explains that she 'looks for people to live in her house who want to be part of a micro-community and not simply rent a room'. 'You want to be able to hang out, chitchat,' she says. 'I want the interaction.' Although the Golden Girls database appears to have closed, other home-share schemes have sprung up.

In Australia, co-housing is becoming a mainstream housing form. Seventy-three-year-old Mary-Faeth Chenery is part of a group of older women in the process of setting up a co-housing project in Daylesford, north-west of Melbourne; it's called WINC – Older Women in Cohousing. It will have a common house, shared guest rooms, a workshop and small individual units.

'It just makes tremendous sense to have a smaller footprint house to save funds that way, but to collaborate with other people who you enjoy being with and help one another,' says Chenery.

Along with the Beguines, I can see in these co-housing models an odd resonance with the concept of the asylum, with micro-communities designed and built around a garden. I'm thinking of the Saint Paul Asylum and Hospital in Saint-Rémy-de-Provence, where in 1889 Vincent van Gogh became a voluntary resident. His painting titled *Garden of the Hospital in Arles*, also known as the *Courtyard of the Hospital at Arles*, shows a formally laid out area with a round central pond from which garden beds radiate outwards, with a tree marking each corner. The garden is framed on four sides by the cloistered walk of the ground floor, with arcade-like galleries above. For Van Gogh, the asylum was a place of order and safety after the disturbing incident in Arles in which he had savagely severed his own ear. Despite bouts of incapacitating illness, the year he spent there was one of his most productive; it resulted in some of his most famous paintings, including *Starry Night*, and the glorious *Blossoming Almond Tree*, a print of which adorns my kitchen wall.

Since Victorian times the word 'asylum' has acquired a taint of madness and incarceration, but in their purest form asylums were places of refuge and retreat, of sanctuary and healing. Designed landscapes were an important feature of 19th-century asylums, as it was believed that tranquil spaces raised the spirits and instilled optimism. And not only were there extensive gardens, but often their care and maintenance were delegated to the patients. As a model, an asylum within a garden, or as part of a farm, can be traced back to the late 18th century in Britain, where it was believed that the institution itself should be part of the therapy.

Is it mad to suggest that these concepts of refuge and retreat, sanctuary and healing, within a garden setting, are precisely the qualities that would best suit us as dwellings in which to live well and age in place? Having evolved into a way of life where so many people – and not only the elderly – find themselves lonely and disconnected, with shrinking familial and social networks, we might logically wish to revive the village model of living.

Some local councils, including my own, are already exploring the possibility of introducing co-housing developments into existing suburbs to accommodate older people who wish to age in place. A preliminary study makes the point that current infill housing, which knocks down one house and replaces it with two or three, increases the density of cities but also the hard-roof and ground-scapes, with a subsequent loss of mature landscape and tree canopies. Houses with smaller footprints and larger communal gardens are better for the environment, and offer the prospect of intergenerational living within a restorative, collectively gardened Eden.

I began by acknowledging that I am privileged to have a garden, and that it is a luxury not available to everyone. And yet, as I write this, I am thinking of the little prince in Antoine de Saint-Exupéry's classic novella, and the single flower he tends on his tiny planet. For the little prince, one flower is sufficient. I'm thinking also of eighty-year-old Philippa, who when she made the decision to move into aged care grieved the loss of her garden. On one of my coffee visits, after describing the sadness of having to walk away from her home and garden, she bravely added: 'My windowsill in my bedroom is full of plants, so that's my little replacement.'

Tending a single pot plant on a balcony or windowsill can bring a daily dose of pleasure to someone with restricted access to nature. There are also community gardens and, having belonged to one for a number of years, I've seen the effect that gardening in company with others can have on those who become involved. Finally, if, or when, a physical garden becomes permanently out of reach, there will always be the possibility of the imagined garden.

Part IV
Spring

No need to hurry. No need to sparkle.
No need to be anybody but oneself.
A Room of One's Own, Virginia Woolf

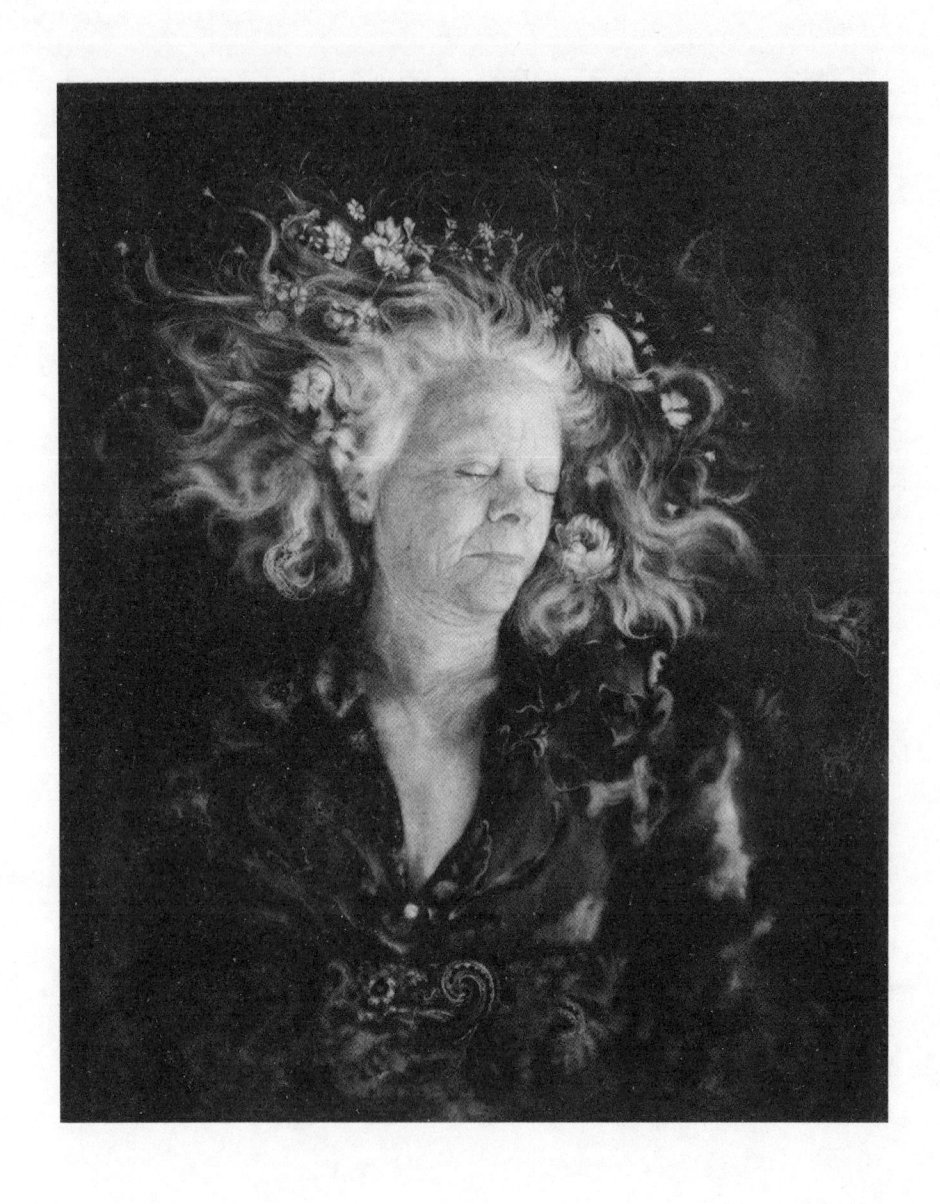

Chapter 15

Imagined Gardens

If the physical garden offers a tangible source of solace, how exquisitely soothing is the imagined garden – and this, I suspect, is where I will spend more time as age diminishes my physical strength. The beauty of such gardens is that there is no need to struggle with unsuitable soil or inhospitable sites. Even weeds may be permanently banished if the gardener so desires. Everything is possible in the imagined garden, and every plant can flourish, even those that are no longer found on earth.

Vita Sackville-West wrote of her plan to create a grey, green and white garden: 'I cannot help hoping that the great ghostly barn-owl will sweep silently across a pale garden, next summer, in the twilight – the pale garden that I am now planting, under the first flakes of snow.' I love that she had that vision, and that she wrote it, and published it, so that we are able to share in its glory. Of course, Vita was by no means all talk, and her white garden at Sissinghurst was dug and planted and is now justly famous, but it existed first in her imagination.

I was introduced to the concept of the imagined garden by the great English garden designer Gertrude Jekyll, who in 1900 wrote about an imaginary wallflower garden. It was to begin with the construction of crumbling walls of just the kind that are 'most esteemed by wall-loving plants'. Jekyll goes on to describe the approach between narrow rock borders planted with light purple aubrietias and two shades of the double cuckoo flower.

Beneath Jekyll's rather formidable exterior lurked not only a poet's soul, but a great writer and imaginer of garden landscapes. Her firm views on colour extended to how best to approach certain parts of the garden. 'Perhaps the grey garden is seen at its best by reaching it through the orange borders.' She described how the strong colour fills and saturates the eye, so that 'standing by the inner yew arch and suddenly turning to look into the grey garden, the effect is surprisingly – quite astonishingly – luminous and refreshing'.

I don't know whether Gertrude Jekyll ever planted her wallflower garden in real life, but, taken by the beauty of her ideas, sometimes at night, with the lights out, I would wander for a while among crumbling masonry and vivid wallflowers. Eventually these entrancing images set me on a path towards imagined gardens of my own, so that now, under Jekyll's influence, I work sometimes in my moon garden. It is a whimsical activity for nights when sleep is elusive, or when I am worried or otherwise agitated. The moon garden is, I suppose, a kind of meditation, but what could be better than to replace one's worries with a visit under a full, or nearly full, moon, to a garden that – if one wants it to be – is always at its peak.

The approach is via a long gravel path, bordered on both sides by the tall, almost mystically elegant sea holly *Eryngium giganteum*, known as 'Miss Willmott's ghost'. I like to think the gravel path would warn of approaching footsteps, since after dark the sight of this haunting plant swaying in the breeze – at five feet, it is, perhaps, just the height of its namesake, Miss Ellen Ann Willmott – could work on fraying nerves.

Ellen Willmott was a horticulturalist of extraordinary passion. Dubbed by Gertrude Jekyll as 'the greatest of all living women gardeners', she used her inherited wealth to establish a legendary garden at Warley, in Essex. The estate, in its heyday, employed up to one hundred gardeners, and was famous for its rivers and drifts and oceans of daffodils – Ellen Willmott had over 600 different species, as well as a notable collection of roses. It was her ambition to create a coloured monograph, *The Genus Rosa*, which would be even more famous than Redouté's *Les Roses*. In pursuit of this dream, she engaged the landscape painter and botanical illustrator Alfred Parsons, a friend of Henry James, to paint her roses. The book, published by John Murray in 1910, was something of a financial disappointment, with only about of a quarter of its copies ever sold.

It was around this time that Willmott's fortune began to decline. While she was collecting honours – being elected to the Royal Horticultural Society's Flora Committee, and receiving a medal from the Royal National Rose Society – she was also arrested in Regent Street on a charge of shoplifting. Having given everything to her gardens, she was now forced to let some of her gardeners go, and to borrow money. The sales of her properties abroad were followed by the sale of family treasures at home, including a Stradivarius violin that Willmott regularly played. Then, during the First World War, the army took over Warley, ruining much of her planting. Old friends died; her maid and travelling companion of twenty years, Lalla Burge, died, and finally Willmott's younger sister Rose succumbed to cancer.

The last decade of Willmott's life was marked by increasing eccentricity, and it was then that the most famous story about her arose: it was said that she would visit the gardens of friends and rivals and, without them knowing, sow the seeds of *Eryngium giganteum*, so that this prickly thistle's blue-white cones, surrounded by wide, silvery bracts, would later emerge in their borders. This is how the plant acquired its common name of Miss Willmott's ghost. She was also reputed to carry a revolver in her handbag when travelling because of a fear that she would be robbed of her jewellery, though by then very little of her jewellery could have remained. Ellen Willmott died alone at Warley on 27 September 1934. Everything that was left was auctioned, and after the war the house was demolished and the garden leased to Essex Naturalists' Trust as a nature reserve – an ignominious end for a once famous and startlingly beautiful garden.

Even now in spring, the rivers and waves and drifts of blue and gold still unfurl across the landscape, and some of her fine old trees remain in the tangled woodland. But Ellen Willmott survives mainly in the many plants that were named after her, in *willmottiae* and *warleyensis* hybrids, including the beautiful *Ceratostigma willmottianum*, or pale blue Chinese plumbago.

From the gravel path, then, a turn through an archway of old brickwork – in which white valerian and the tiny star-faced seaside daisy spring from cracks and crevices – leads into my moon garden. Since scent is vital in a garden that will be visited at night, the long borders are crammed with night-scented stocks, white tobacco flowers, gardenias and the pale trumpets of perfumed lilies. Star jasmine might spring to mind for some gardeners, but for me its heavy odour overpowers other, more delicate scents. There are masses of roses and, here and there, sometimes even in the pathways, double white hollyhocks have been allowed to self-seed; it is the same with white borage, and the white cosmos 'Purity', which is known as a windflower. As the curving backdrop to a pond that reflects the stars, I am nurturing a hedge of the Australian native *Telopea speciosissima* 'Wirrimbirra White', the rare white waratah. There is almost no end to what could be planted in this night garden. Grey- and silver-leaved plants must be included, of course, to make the white flowers appear even more luminous under the moon.

In her autobiographical novel *Spinster*, Sylvia Ashton-Warner creates the character of Anna Vorontosov, the genius teacher of little Māori children in a remote New Zealand town, a passionate woman who in her spare time nurtures a blue garden. 'I notice the delphiniums. They make me think of men. The way they bloom so hotly in the summer, then die right out of sight in the winter, only to push up mercilessly again when the growth starts, is like my memory of love.' She likens the intense blue of the flowers to distilled passion. In a book structured by the seasons, Anna writes that in summer her flowers are 'all chatter and flash. And the funny thing is that you never hear them talk about the spring before, much less the autumn to come. And as for winter! They wouldn't know how to say the word.'

Gertrude Jekyll's plans for a blue garden are rather more staid and strict than Anna's, though still beautiful. While she does not allow purple-blues – 'they would not be admissible' – she does allow a few of the palest yellow flowers (snapdragons) and the 'foam-white', the 'milk-white' and the 'almond-white' (clematis and lupins) that make her blue plants appear all the bluer. Jekyll considers Miss Willmott's ghost admissible, a nod to the horticulturalist who visited the great plants-woman in her own garden at Munstead.

The French writer Colette, whose books were full of botanical detail, did not cease gardening even when age and arthritis kept her bedridden. At night, in her rooms in the Palais-Royal, Colette roamed imagined gardens. 'There is nothing so terrible about not having a garden any more. The worrying thing would be if the future garden, whose reality is of no importance, were beyond my grasp. But it is not.' Colette plans her 'tomorrow garden', specifying pansies 'with wide faces, beards, and moustaches – that look like Henry VIII'. Nothing is too difficult for the imaginative gardener. 'An arbour? Naturally I shall have an arbour. I'm not down to my last arbour yet.'

Physical gardening tires me more quickly than it once did, yet still I send away for packets of special seed. This winter I ordered Miss Jekyll's cuckoo flower (otherwise known as lady's smock, mayflower, or milkmaids), thinking to give it a try, even though it may not much care for a South Australian summer. I sow, and pot on, and plant out. I even maintain a vegetable plot in a nearby community garden. But there are many nights before sleep when I linger in imagined gardens.

As well as the moon garden there is a walled apothecary, beds of medicinal plants edged with black pansy borders. I am building this little by little, using the language of *Culpeper's Complete Herbal & English Physician*. The wild there being better than the tame, this is a place where blowsy roses ramble unchecked over sheds and walls, a garden whose medicinal heart is enclosed within an outer layer of thorny yet romantic disorder.

Plants in this garden fall under government and virtues. The 'wild parsnip', for example, is under Venus. It is a plant that resists and remedies the biting of serpents, eases the pains and stitches in the sides, and dissolves wind in both the stomach and the bowel. All plums, too, are under Venus, but my beloved quince trees are owned by Saturn. The juice of the quince, taken in small quantities, is of great efficacy in sicknesses, vomiting, eructations and purgings. Quinces, when they are green, help all sorts of fluxes; the mucilaginous seeds in water make an excellent medicine for sore mouths.

Nicholas Culpeper is another of gardening's legendary characters. Born in 1616 in Surrey, the son of a vicar, Nicholas excelled at Cambridge and was expected to enter either the church or medicine. However, his life took a bizarre turn when he fell hopelessly in love. Having borrowed £200 from his mother, he arranged to meet his beloved under a prominent oak tree near Lewes. On the night of their elopement, he galloped from Cambridge through a lashing storm only to find that the oak had been struck by lightning and his love lay dead. Shattered by this loss, Culpeper almost gave in to despair. He was eventually persuaded by his parents to take up an apothecary position in London. In 1640 he started his own practice in Red Lion Street, Spitalfields, which at that time teemed with the poor, the sick, the dispossessed.

In those days, doctors held a protectionist view of the medical profession; they kept their knowledge to themselves, though it was beyond the reach of ordinary people. Doctors looked down on apothecaries as ignorant druggists, though they were the only form of health care the poor could afford. Culpeper began his work for the needy of London by translating the *London Pharmacopoeia of the College of Physicians* from

Latin into English, calling it the *London Dispensatory*. Then, in 1653, he published his great herbal, *The English Physician*, a comprehensive and practical guide to herbal medicine, which has remained in print ever since. I love Culpeper both for his devotion to the needs of London's poor and for the beauty of the language of his herbal, which is the language of Shakespeare.

In delving into the ways we humans develop new habits, I came across the phrase 'embodied semantics'. This is a process in which brain connectivity during a thought-about action mirrors the connectivity that occurs during the actual action – for example, thinking about running can trigger some of the same neural connections as physically running. Habitual negativity, I learned, rewires the brain, and ultimately damages it by shrinking the hippocampus – one of the main areas that is destroyed by Alzheimer's disease.

Bringing these ideas together made me wonder whether a positive habit, such as imagining a garden, could rewire one's brain in a good way. Might such repeated activity offset the effects of stress and heal long-term grief? Might it be so restorative that it could slow, or even arrest, the decline of the age-altered brain?

Looking back over my years, it is as if I am seeing satellite images of once-lush landscapes in the wake of various storms: there are definite areas of wreckage; scattered debris. Sometimes I see the years as a heaving ocean with only a few tiny time-islands of calm abiding. I dread what remains of my life becoming more chaotic. I have never been able to meditate; a yoga practice has never held me for long, and I do not sleep well. So how am I to change my brain, to steer it calmly and with dignity into and through old age? Gardens have always been places of refuge, so with nothing to lose and everything to gain, and, it must be admitted, with no better plan, I am placing my faith in the restorative rewiring of these garden imaginings.

As the need arises, there will be further gardens. Already I plan a Garden of Lost Flowers, to give sanctuary to such beauties as *Medusagyne oppositifolia*, a jellyfish tree endemic to the island of Mahé in the Seychelles, and *Viola cryana*, the cry violet, or cry pansy, an extinct plant species that was once endemic to Yonne. The Garden Where Nothing Is Forgotten and All Is Forgiven must, I think, be a blue garden, though one in which the purple-blues will be admissible.

Inspiration comes from all corners of the earth, but especially from the real-life gardening and garden writing of wonderful gardeners like Edna Walling, who was so influential in Australia, and Gertrude Jekyll, who as well as being a great designer and plants-woman was a fearless writer and imaginer of gardens. And thanks to Miss Jekyll, and to Vita Sackville-West, any of us can wander among crumbling masonry and vivid wallflowers, or drift towards sleep on the barn owl's silent swoop across a pale summer garden.

In the months to come, when summer settles on the garden, I will yearn for the lushness of these weeks when the green is almost acidic in its brightness. As the month begins it is still a time of anticipation. Buds are swelling on the rose bushes; I am weeding and trying to bring some sense of order to the tangle of plants in the places I allowed to go wild through last summer and autumn. My final flourish, once space is created, is to arrange for a delivery of cottage mulch.

For a week or so, the mulch makes the garden look like an exemplary, weed-free place, where all is kept under tight control. But this doesn't last. Soon the weeds poke through – this is the time to pounce on them, when they are weakened by effort. But although I do my best, many of them quietly take hold again. They do this because I am distracted by the progress of the roses. I spend too much time watching them to see which will be the first of the season to bloom.

Extract from my garden journal, September 2021

Chapter 16

Russian Dolls and Roses

While sorting through old papers, I turn up a letter I wrote to my mother. It is postmarked 16 February 1995. On bright yellow paper, it is from another country – the Isle of Man – but it might as well be from another planet. On that planet, a woman like me but twenty-five years younger has been making green velvet curtains by hand, painstakingly stitching lining and inter-lining according to instructions in a book on curtain-making by Caroline Clifton-Mogg. Last thing at night, the woman has gone into the room where she has been sewing all day, to gloat over her handiwork. She has picked up one of the almost finished curtains to give it a stroke, and found *the velvet pile is running the wrong way. I've made it upside down!* Even at this great distance, I feel her pain.

The woman writes that her ten-year-old daughter is to play her flute in the school concert, that she draws a lovely sound from the difficult instrument. Crocuses are flowering in her garden, and she is looking forward to peonies and poppies. In Australia, her mother has planted, or plans to plant, black tulips. The woman plays in a band, and earlier that evening the drummer has rung to say they've been asked to play a charity gig for a sick child. They will, of course, she writes, even though it is on a school night. She has made curtains for her daughter's bedroom – peach damask – and she dreams of making a mixed star patchwork quilt. *Greens are my colours at the moment*, she writes, despite the upset with the velvet curtains.

How well I know that kitchen where she sits at the sturdy scrubbed table to write to her mother. I still have the table, the chairs, the flute, but not the daughter who played it so sweetly. The drummer is gone to pancreatic cancer. For all I know the green velvet may still hang in the hall window of that lovely house; some textiles endure for decades, especially velvet.

When my envy subsides, it is replaced by a stab of pity for this woman: it is clear she has no clue how her life will play out. She cannot see me as I see her – still energetic, still optimistic, not yet wounded, not yet bitterly counting her sorrows and losses, nor the aches and pains of her body as it gradually accommodates the wear and tear of age. Although she writes from a country where she was always cold, seen from this distance she inhabits a perpetual summertime – this woman with her mass of henna-bright hair.

The question I ask as I fold the letter away is whether I still carry this woman inside, and, yes, some days I feel that young woman close to the surface – like a face at a window, indistinct behind net curtains. On other days I cannot catch even a glimpse; she has stepped away from the window into the murk of lost time. But the woman at the window is only one of many selves. They flicker, will-o'-the-wisp-like, in peripheral vision, or they emerge, clear-voiced, from the pages of old letters and journals. For the most part, though, they remain hidden, Russian dolls nested in memory.

Perhaps it is the damp, or the cooler nights, but I am stiff and slow-moving these mornings. As I totter to the kitchen to make the first cup of tea of the day, I feel every year of my age, yet within minutes of setting out on my daily walk the long muscles in my back and legs begin to stretch, and I move more fluidly. It is vital to maintain this daily walking routine, which I am ashamed to admit I only started after my first visit to a cardiologist.

One morning, in the spring before last, I woke before daylight to find my heart beating too fast, and in a weird and ungainly rhythm. In the darkness it felt surreal, and I decided I must be dreaming. But my eyes were open, and when I touched the pulse at my wrist it was both ragged and rapid. I tried calming thoughts, deep breathing. I rose and drank a glass of water. Nothing worked.

While I waited for the doctor's surgery to open, I looked out at the softness of the early morning garden. Rose bushes were forming buds; tiny quince leaves looked like bright green bows tied to the branches and the new plum trees were stirring into life. I wondered, self-dramatising, if I would live to see the new rose and the clematis in flower. It seems maudlin now, but at the time my heart felt like it might fail at any moment. I realised it had been beating every minute of every hour since the day I was born, which was a long time ago. Why had I imagined it would never tire?

Everything in the garden seemed unbearably frail and lovely that morning, and I never wanted to look away. Through all of this the blackbird sang in the jacaranda tree – long, pensive, exquisite solos. His song was so pure it brought tears to my eyes, and I could well understand how the early settlers longed to hear his familiar fluting whistle in this new land. I thought of the pairs of imported birds, their wretched existence during long sea voyages, caged in the stuffy holds of sailing ships along with other livestock. How those early birds must have wondered at the strangeness of everything when at last they were released – trees, sky, heat, the new fragrances of native vegetation. Did their repertoire alter as a result of this abrupt change, or did they carry on singing their ancestral songs?

That morning as I listened to the blackbird, it seemed that every time he reached the end of a phrase another bird would sing it back to him from further away. And then another, more distant still, repeated the second bird's song. It went beyond the range of my hearing, but for a moment I had a vision of the early morning city with its gardens stitched together by birdsong.

After my appointment with the cardiologist, I began daily walking; I lost what he described as 'a therapeutic amount' of weight, and adopted a low-cholesterol diet. Exercise was the important thing, the cardiologist said, though it was not something the drug companies ever promoted.

At a follow-up appointment I was sent for an echocardiogram, and on the technician's screen saw the mitral valve of my heart at work.

'It looks like a tiny hand in there, waving,' I said.

The operator turned a startled face. 'Yes!' she said. 'So it does.'

In Kate Llewellyn's memoir *A Fig at the Gate*, she stresses the importance of exercise. 'It's walk or die!' Kate insists, and I believe her. Walk or die! I mutter on these damp mornings when to lie in bed late seems a more attractive option.

Kate writes that at sixty she thought that when she was seventy she would be entering old age. 'Now that I am seventy I think, "When I am eighty I will be old."' This is how she tricks herself into delaying old age, a strategy enabled by her robust health.

Before Covid came, there was a weekend when we travelled to Melbourne. It was all about the beloved boy and his football team, but for me there was a certain amount of culture shock: where once I would have enjoyed the big city buzz, in the midst of it I found myself craving silence, and the calming stillness of my garden.

In our hotel opposite Fitzroy Gardens, people passed through reception, through the bar and restaurant, in a constant stream; they entered and exited the lifts. Modern life is restless, and establishments like the one we stayed at are geared to cope with the relentless traffic. Melbourne's trams, with their quaint *ting-ting*, evoked the atmosphere of an earlier era, but on board there was a crush of people, exuding odours of perfume, pizza, smoke-soaked clothing.

At night, struggling to sleep in our overheated hotel room, I visualised our empty rooms at home, their impassive silence. I thought, too, of the darkened garden, the cosmos flowers swaying at the slightest breath of air, the laden quince trees, the curves of their fruit picked out here and there by starlight. I imagined the dark angel on her plinth, head and wings melting into the night, and I thought of the Elizabeth Bishop poem 'Questions of Travel', in which she wonders whether it might have been better to have stayed at home, and only thought of the destination.

When at last we flew home it felt to me like waking with a dream still fresh. The ornamental pears that were turning colour when we left were a vivid shade of plum, and each one was surrounded by a shed petticoat of leaves. It looked like autumn, yet the weather was warm. I poached quinces and baked quince cake, and picked the last of the roses; I sat on the veranda for hours, soaking it all in: home.

Waking the next morning, I was relieved to hear the magpie's fluting call and the rumble of the 172 bus in place of Melbourne's constant roar. There, apart from some sparrows scouting for biscuit crumbs at the outdoor cafes, I had not been aware of the presence of birds. I was happy to be home, yet there was an initial strangeness, too, a faint coolness, as if the house was putting us in our place – Oh, there you are! I thought you had gone for good.

As I work in the garden, that yellow letter sends out ripples across the surface of my mind. I find myself lamenting that, although hurriedly written and on any old paper, it conjures a life more vivid than the one I am currently living. The voice of the letter is also unmistakably my own, perhaps more so than anything I have written since. Is this because it was intended for one specific, much-loved reader? Has everything I've written in the interim – and I have written a lot – been too self-conscious, too confused about its readership? I soothe myself with the thought that not everything I have written has missed the mark: there is that slender book in which I managed to squeeze almost my entire life into little more than 150 pages.

In *The Happiness Glass* I unfolded the life of a fictional character, Lily Brennan. Lily is both me and not me; mostly she is a series of younger versions of me, the Russian dolls unpacked, the me of perpetual summertime, the me of seasons still to come. In it I take Lily from her outback childhood to her widowed late sixties, where she is in a nursing home following a minor stroke. The interesting thing about that final story has been the reaction of friends, who have told me they didn't care for it because they didn't want to imagine me (or perhaps themselves) in the aged-care environment. In writing Lily's life, I was exploring both what *had* happened and what I feared *might* happen. Perhaps I hoped to exorcise my nursing home dread by first trying it out in fiction. In the final story, Lily will not stay if it is possible to leave. Was I reassuring myself that whatever befalls me I will still be capable of planning and executing an escape?

Longstanding friendships between women form the core of Charlotte Wood's novel *The Weekend*. In it, old friends Jude, Wendy and Adele – all in their seventies – arrive at the beach house of their late friend Sylvie to clear the property ahead of its sale. The three women have been successful in their chosen fields – Jude in the upmarket restaurant trade, Wendy as a public intellectual and academic, Adele as an actress – but their glory days are waning, and in Adele's case, once the weekend is over she looks set to become homeless.

The behind-the-scenes bitchiness, the shifting allegiances and exasperated affection of those who know each other well accurately portray friendship, despite the unwavering, steady-as-a-torch-beam narrative of long-term friendship we would prefer to believe. The truth is that we are often irritated by our friends, even though we love them. And which non-dog-lover hasn't inwardly groaned when a pal has turned up with a large and grubby-looking specimen in tow? Thus it is with Jude and Wendy, and Wendy's ancient dog Finn. Finn, who in dog years is more ancient than the women, becomes a focus of attention for each of them, and you could say he is made to bear too much of the weight of the women's fear and loathing of their own ageing.

And loathe it they do, though each woman in her own way remains hopeful of something good still to come. For Wendy it is her work, and the ideas for a new book she senses will soon crystallise. Jude is looking forward to spending time with her long-term, married lover once the house clearing is over. Adele, out of work and at the end of her latest relationship, settles her faith firmly in something turning up, as it always has done. But acting is an unforgiving profession, and she is humiliated for her fantasy of 'clawing back her one great moment on the stage, from thirty years ago' when we see her through the eyes of the arrogant young director Joe Gillespie. 'Gillespie was not dancing with Adele but laughing at her ... a pissed old luvvie spilling out of her clothes'. Joe is recording Adele dancing on his phone. 'You old girls are fucking hilarious.'

Could anything be more painful? And yet there is worse to come. The tensions of the weekend break open a long-kept secret, a betrayal that involves a betrayal. Despite the chaos that engulfs them, old friendships somehow hold. But by the end of the book two of the three face uncertain futures, and *The Weekend*'s portrayal of older women does not instil confidence.

On the internet, I read an interview with Doris Lessing in which she confesses to a lingering nostalgia for her younger self. I make a note to return to this, but when I do, after hours of searching, I can no longer find the website. Eventually I begin to think I must have imagined it, or that I had been pondering the question of the younger self we carry inside us while reading Doris writing as Jane Somers in the *Diary of a Good Neighbour*.

In that book, the fierce old woman Maudie Fowler carries her younger self inside, though her outer appearance is of a tiny, bent-over woman 'with a nose nearly meeting her chin, in black heavy dusty clothes, and something not far off a bonnet'. The rooms Maudie lives in, too, have a daunting appearance, yet she will not consider moving, or even having helpers. 'With your own place,' Maudie says, 'you've got everything. Without it, you are a dog. You are nothing.'

When the narrator, Janna, calls in a young electrician to fix Maudie's faulty light, he says, shocked at the state of the place, 'Why isn't she in a Home? She shouldn't be living like that.' Janna answers, 'She doesn't want to go into a Home. She likes it where she is.' But the electrician, Jim, is troubled by Maudie. 'What's the good of people that old?' he says. And then, quickly, to cancel out what he was thinking, 'Well, we'll be old one of these days, I suppose.' Of course, Lessing is behind Jim the electrician's response, and she gives him that moment of realisation. But in real life not everyone reaches the same conclusion, obvious though it is, because if they did surely ageist thinking would seem absurd.

A personal experience of ageism burns itself into the memory; it is not easily forgotten, or forgiven. Lately I have been noticing smaller moments, when ageism surfaces unconsciously. Like last weekend, during a seed saving and propagation workshop at the community garden, when the thirty-something tutor remarked that he had only recently relaxed his tough stance against plants that cannot be eaten. He casually, and rather scathingly, linked 'ornamentals' with 'people older than me' for whom he works as a gardener.

While he blithered on, oblivious, I thought about my own garden – its gentle, meditative quality in almost any season makes me noticeably less stressed; it slows my heart rate (and I am certain of this because my watch tracks it). Although at first glance it might appear merely decorative, it is fenced by productive fruit trees, and the roses are under-planted with herbs, many of which are edible. Others are medicinal – they will help you sleep, they will bind your wounds, and one or two could kill you. The whole garden is a good strong medicine, to be taken in through the eyes and ears and nose and, sometimes, with caution, the mouth. I could even, if I so desired, eat the roses.

As I write this, still nettled, that bloke is three days older than when he inadvertently revealed his ageist mindset. And going forward he will only get older still, because there is no way back for any of us. Already, likely without realising, he carries a younger version of himself inside. The thing to wonder is how much time will pass before he reaches an awareness that age happens to us only if we are lucky. And how much more time before he, too, finds himself in urgent need of a rose.

These evenings when the light is green, and the shadows, too, are green, and the first crickets begin their creaking chant, I'm inclined to feel immortal. It's to do with the garden's sense of timelessness, knowing that other gardeners down the centuries have experienced this same feeling of being held suspended in the sweet soft breath of early spring.

Extract from my garden journal, September 2021

Chapter 17

The Ordinary and Extraordinary

I am standing on the footpath outside our house looking up into a jacaranda tree when a flock of corellas passes over. In the tawny late-afternoon light their white-feathered bodies shimmer and shine like souls migrating; they are noisy in flight – whether from joy, or fright, or to keep the flock together, I have no idea – but the sight of this cloud of restless spirits plunges in through my eyes like a sword of light. It is a vision from childhood, a memory laid down in the past's bottom-most layers. When a second wave of birds follows, all shrieking urgently, the air heaves like the ocean, its running tide of feathers a glorious whirling white fused with the sky's tremulous, immortal blue. They beat away towards the coast, leaving me refreshed by the beauty of their passage. I watch until they have vanished, and when I turn, I see that there are people passing who have not noticed this spectacle; they are not looking up but down.

It is hard to hold in one's mind the preciousness of the ordinary, for we are as fish in water. We may pay lip-service to mindfulness, but in the impatient and distracting world most of us inhabit, how closely do we attend to all the small yet matchless moments in a day, when we exist, if we but realised, in a kind of earthly paradise. A walk to the cafe in spring sunshine to meet a friend for coffee; to sit with a book and enter a world laid out for our pleasure upon crisp cream pages; closing one's eyes to sleep in a quiet room, free from pain and looking forward to the new day: how often do we note such moments in our diaries?

Because there will come a morning when some turn of events sweeps all of this away. There will be a phone call, or a letter, or the result of a blood test, and it is then, suddenly, that we will understand the value of ordinary days. As we fret for them to be returned to us, prayers may be wrung out in the silence after lights out, extravagant bargains proffered. Sometimes the universe will answer, but mostly it will shrug.

So I watch the corellas pass over, and what I wish for is an angel. I have in mind a being like the one that kneels beside the Virgin Mary in Leonardo da Vinci's *Madonna of the Rocks*, serene yet capable, with soft-feathered wings and one of the most exquisite faces ever painted. And if I should ever stumble upon a giant's purse containing a magic golden bean, or if my sleeve should brush against a lamp and a genie emerges to grant me a single wish, it will be this: that Leonardo's angel cup her hands around my ordinary days.

~

Back in 2017, my world lurched sideways while I was at the hairdresser's. I had felt fine when I walked in, but in the time it took to cut and blow-dry my hair I began to feel dizzy. Leaving the salon, I staggered like a drunken sailor; in the parking lot I had to hold on to a wall to remain upright. At home, stricken with dizziness and nausea, I might have thought I was having a stroke if another family member hadn't experienced the same symptoms only a few days earlier. After two hours their dizziness had passed, as it did for me, so I guessed that we'd had a virus, and there was little to be done but rest. A week later, my symptoms returned, though not so severely. I was left with post-viral fatigue, and a blocked ear.

But sometime later, with the ear still giving trouble, an audiologist found significant hearing loss. By now there was also intermittent and terrible tinnitus, which for someone who adores silence was beyond tormenting. The clatter of a busy cafe, once so companionable, now caused discomfort, a condition known as hyperacusis. When walking I often felt light-headed, and an ear, nose and throat specialist diagnosed viral labyrinthitis. The virus had invaded my inner ear, he said, and the damage to my hearing would be permanent.

But asymmetrical hearing loss raises various suspicions, and before I knew it I was in the waiting room for an MRI scan. I'd gone from a cut and blow-dry to a possible brain tumour.

~

Leonardo da Vinci painted the *Madonna of the Rocks* twice, with minor differences. One picture hangs in the National Gallery in London, while the other is in the Louvre. Debate still rages over which was painted first, but both pictures depict the Virgin Mary, the infant Jesus and John the Baptist as a baby, as well as the kneeling angel. The cave-like setting was considered eccentric when it was painted, and it is thought by one Vincian scholar to relate to Leonardo's experience in a cave in the Italian countryside.

There are variations of colour and light between the two works, but the most striking differences are in the angel – in the Parisian version her robes are red and green, her finger points to one of the infants, and her calm yet knowing gaze is directed towards the viewer. The London angel wears soft blue robes; her hand rests quietly on her knee, and her lowered eyelids give her face a contemplative though dream-charged expression.

In 2005, using infrared reflectography, the London painting was found to have a pentimento, the traces of an earlier image underneath. A woman, most likely kneeling, with her right hand outstretched and her left on her heart, was discovered, as if Leonardo had planned another pose for the angel, and then changed his mind.

Reflectography sounds like something Leonardo da Vinci might have invented. He would surely have been fascinated by infrared light's capacity to render layers of paint transparent and reveal the under-drawing. It works because black pigments, such as graphite and charcoal, absorb the infrared rays and become visible. The technique was developed in the 1960s by a Dutch physicist to improve upon the earlier infrared photography, in which blue and green pigments remain opaque. In reflectography the painting is lit by infrared light, and an infrared-sensitive camera captures the light reflected back from the surface of the painting. When this reflection is digitised by a computer, what lies beneath the paint appears on the screen in black and white.

The process strikes me as close to the exchange of light between painting and viewer: the searching gaze of a great work of art acts as both light source and camera, and in response to its radiance we reflect back our pentimenti. In the context of art the Italian verb *pentirsi*, to repent, seems to imply that the creation of a great painting has a spiritual dimension, confessional in some way, and redemptive. In the context of humans, and the revelations that can be drawn through close observation of works of art, our pentimenti may consist of anything from remnants of our younger selves to lost loves, old griefs, unrealised dreams, the traces of exploratory excursions along roads not taken.

Whatever my personal under-drawing once was, there are times now when I fancy that the image that lies beneath the London Madonna, of the woman with her hand outstretched, is not so different from my current pentimento: prodded from dormancy when the world goes suddenly awry, with one hand she clutches at her heart, and with the other implores the universe.

~

I find it moving that when a knife-wielding intruder invaded his home in the middle of the night, the Beatle George Harrison chanted 'Hare Krishna, Hare Krishna' as he lunged forward to fight for his life. It was almost twenty years after John Lennon was fatally shot, when an obsessed fan, thirty-four-year-old Michael Abram, somehow breached the security of Harrison's Oxfordshire home. With stab wounds, and the walls and carpet splashed with blood, George and his wife Olivia believed they were about to die. That the musician invoked Krishna at such a moment proved that of the four Beatles who went to India in the late sixties, for George Harrison it was more than a passing dalliance with a famous guru.

Few of us know what we will blurt out in a crisis. The words we reach for may not make sense in any other part of our lives. For example, there have been times of great darkness, even terror, when I have found myself clinging to some remembered lines from Psalm 23. I am not a churchgoer, or even a believer, so this is the residue of a childhood in which the maternal side of my family went to church on Sundays and read the bible on other days of the week. But even to a non-believer Psalm 23 in the King James Version is compelling in its rhythms, and the language, stripped to its beautiful bones, enters the ear like music.

Yea, though I walk through the valley of the shadow of death, I will fear no evil: it is quite some mantra, and although it may be useless to protect against mania, somehow its simple beauty bolsters courage. And how often and unexpectedly in life we find ourselves on the crumbling path above that menacing abyss. The psalm's gentle imagery is the stuff of untroubled days; in its green pastures and still waters, if we need to be reminded, our *cup runneth over*. The final lines draw us in towards their shepherded safety: *Surely goodness and mercy shall follow me all the days of my life...* those old writers – those psalmists who lived through biblical wars, and storms, and plagues – they knew that the still, green days were the ones worth savouring.

~

So I entered the place where a scan would be made of my brain. It was the Valley of the Shadow of Death if I ever saw it: a room of hard shiny surfaces and bulky machines, and with a small side room in which I would undress and put on a blue robe made of a kind of dishcloth material. The control room where the technicians sat was dim, but in the scanning room the lights beamed cold and bright; I lay stretched on a table in my flimsy robe, as exposed as one of those blind white curl grubs I dig up in the garden. To communicate my dread of this procedure perhaps I should disclose that not only my darling father died of a brain tumour but also his younger brother. I tell myself that the female side of the family is strong, and they are, but that nagging voice in my ear whispers that the division of genes is unpredictable.

Lying within the MRI machine's heavy presence, my head cradled in a skull-shaped dish, I was offered headphones with the option of radio to block the noise of the scanner. But what if I was immobilised while in the grip of some song that afterwards I would not be able to stop singing, as once, for one terrible week, I could not stop singing the song of the Collingwood Football Club? Rather than risk it, I opted for silence.

Having my head clamped in place caused a passing panic, but worse than this was the thought of what those magnetic waves might sketch on the screen in the control room. The machine's gaze would be pitiless, I knew, penetrating skin and bone to scour the caverns and crevasses of the brain, a cold, withholding light, lacking art's redemptive radiance. A mirror angled above my head showed me that the world was now upside down. The scanner began a terrible grinding noise, and then, without having planned it, I summoned in my head the sound of John Lennon singing 'Across the Universe'. The detail I could bring to it was astonishing: I even had the sliding acoustic guitar chords of the intro.

How can we know, until such moments, what is really inside us? Henri Matisse famously declared that he was made of all that he had seen, but it would appear that we are made of all that we have heard and read as well.

As the scan progressed, with its unearthly sounds, I held to the mantra-like lyrics that Lennon claimed were the best he ever wrote. They came, he said, in a flow from somewhere, as if they had already been composed and were being delivered. I dare not reproduce them here, for the rights to quote song lyrics are some of the most difficult permissions to obtain. But the melodic line of 'Across the Universe' is long and flowing, and it contains the mantra *Jai guru deva Om*, a Sanskrit fragment that translates approximately as 'glory to the shining remover of darkness'.

The song begins with an endless flow of words across the universe, an image bound to appeal to a writer. The final stanza brings the message of the limitless undying love that shines around us ... surely a sixties-style cosmic echo of Psalm 23. In the circumstances, it was the perfect distraction, and as the scan ground on I ran through it over and over, wondering what kind of brain activity might be mapped by my silent singing.

Later, walking towards the comfort of an Italian restaurant where I would order salty schiacciata and a glass of good red wine, I thought about how effortlessly art acts as 'the shining remover of darkness', and that this, without doubt, is what art is for.

Resting on the veranda at dusk, I notice the heart shape made by two parrots sitting close together in the jacaranda tree. Suddenly the blackbird swoops in and perches above, unleashing wild trills in the failing light.

My quince trees in their twelfth summer surge skywards with the boundless energy of sleek young dogs or prancing ponies. I am proud to have been the one who planted those quinces, though I will not see them when they are half a century old and much less supple. By then their stately trunks and limbs – so carefully tended in the important early years by Peter the tree pruner – will be more beautifully patinated. The young man who shares my garden might see them, though.

Lately I have begun to think of planting more for him than for myself. I am considering starting some slow-growing box, shapes that will mature alongside him, so that at dusk on some distant evening, as a grown man, or even an old one, he might sit on this same veranda in the fading light and feel my love for him as a continuing presence.

Extract from my garden journal, October 2021

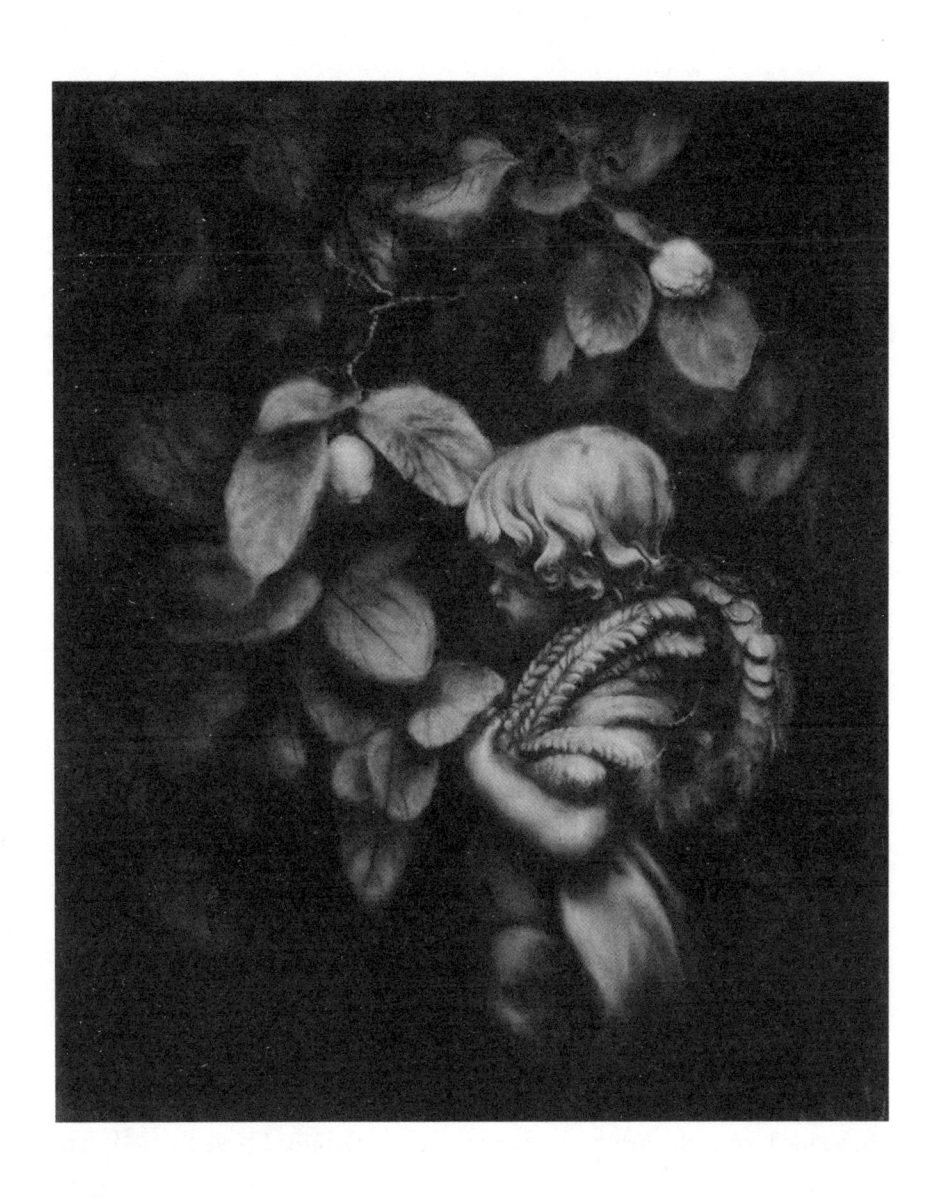

Chapter 18

The Homeward Star

> O Evening Star, bringing everything
> that dawn's first glimmer scattered far and wide –
> You bring the sheep, you bring the goat,
> You bring the child back to the mother.
>
> Fragment 104, Sappho

Writers and artists have always responded to twilight's mystery. Sometimes, as with Colette's *L'Étoile Vesper*, it provides a late-life motif for a backward-glancing book. Sometimes a response seems to inadvertently offer an unguarded glimpse of the writer, as in the last published piece of the great Victorian artist, art critic and writer John Ruskin, in which he recalls the cry of a corncrake at dusk in the fields above his home, Brantwood. 'Twilight after twilight I have hunted that bird, and never once got glimpse of it: the voice was always at the other side of the field, or in the inscrutable air or earth.'

Whether it is a lit window seen from a darkened garden in the twilight paintings of the French artist Henri Le Sidaner, or an etching by the 19th-century British painter and printmaker Samuel Palmer of a shepherd gathering in his flock, artists across time have portrayed dusk as a gathering place of our vulnerabilities, our memories and yearnings.

Writers, too, have addressed its nostalgic quality. In 1968, the novelist William Maxwell wrote to Sylvia Townsend Warner of the long summer evenings in rural Ireland. They are, he said, like 'having everything you had ever lost given back to you'. Maxwell saw this as a boon, yet there are times when having something returned can be more troubling than having it taken away – I am thinking of the hundreds of letters that my mother saved during the decades I lived away from Australia. When I finally came back to settle, she returned them to me. Three old brown leather suitcases, stuffed with scrambled despatches from the many places I had lived: a motley archive, I thought, yet for a writer it was gold.

Without even opening the letters I could see that they contained so much more than the sometimes hastily scrawled news of my whereabouts. The bulging envelopes, with their often-exquisite foreign stamps, the thin blue aerogram pages, had preserved decades of forgotten detail, which I found I was strangely reluctant to recall. It would be more than fifteen years before I mustered the will to put them in order. Occasionally I would open one of the suitcases and be appalled by the mess. I fancied faint sounds issued from the torn-open envelopes. They had a wounded look that made me think of some lines from Joan Didion's *Slouching Towards Bethlehem*: 'We forget all too soon the things we thought we could never forget. We forget the loves and the betrayals alike, forget what we whispered and what we screamed, forget who we were.'

The letters contained some of what I had whispered and a little of what I had screamed, along with a good part of who I had once been. Why I thought sorting through them would be an ideal occupation in the early days of the Covid crisis is beyond me. I know it struck me that if I caught the virus and died, no one would ever make sense of their chaos. Why that even mattered, I cannot say, but somehow in that first shocked moment of realisation that everyday life as we knew it had changed, and not for the good, it seemed imperative in the chaotic present to impose order on the chaotic past.

Easter 2020 was a different world from the one in which I had once hidden chocolate eggs in various nooks in the garden. When I wasn't spraying disinfectant on household surfaces, on car door handles and steering wheels, when I wasn't rationing rolls of toilet paper, or nerving myself to broach the supermarket, I was sitting on the floor of my study surrounded by hundreds of tattered envelopes. They were the dried husks of years lived as richly and unconsciously as flowers bloom and wither, the seeds of a life, dispersed on the wind, and diligently collected by my mother.

It appeared I'd had a habit of never dating my letters. Sourly I reflected that this was probably because I was so flaky that I literally never knew what day it was. I think I was harsh on myself, because there weren't the devices we rely on now to remind us of such things, and, in those far-off times, young women making their way did not invest in calendars. Perhaps time was even different then: I have the impression that it moved more slowly. While I may not have been fussy about the date, I always noted my address. Because the fact of *having* an address was often the most important feature of my precarious and shiftless life, especially in the early years, when at twenty-one I had left Australia. The addresses allowed me to track my progress with reasonable accuracy across that wilderness of years. I sorted the letters into bundles: New Zealand; South Africa; London; East Sussex; Australia; Chile; the Isle of Man. And then into sub-sections of the addresses I had moved to within those locations.

I tried not to get sidetracked from the sorting by reading, but some letters were without their envelopes, or there would be a stray page I needed to scan to identify where it belonged. The sight of some of those letters shivered through me like an electric shock: I remembered where I was when they were written, saw a younger self, sealing the envelope and licking the stamps – sometimes it was impossible not to open them and dive in.

Photographs slithered out into my lap, or newspaper cuttings. The moment I freed a letter and smoothed its pages flat, it felt like a driving instructor had taken over the steering in one of those dual-control cars. I was gripped by the lost worlds these missives unfolded. They contained all the big stuff – births, deaths, marriages – but also the minutia, the ordinary material that makes up the bulk of our lives.

In the mornings, dodging other walkers and trying not to touch anything, wondering whether even the breeze posed a threat, and bereft that I could not reward myself with coffee because my favourite cafe was closed, its lovely baristas stood down, my vision would blur and I would be forced to stop. I wept, leaning against brush fences or under sheltering trees; it was a slow but inexorable welling of grief. I felt anxious for my mother in her extreme old age, for the young man in my care who was not yet eighteen, and for my immunocompromised beloved. I felt anxious for myself, too, but there was also the almost unbearable weight of those letters – they filled three plastic storage boxes; I had decanted them from the dusty suitcases.

I began to realise that there could be important reasons for forgetting, not the least of them that crowding the events of those years into my present was seriously destabilising. The letters clamoured with the names of the dead, friends who had been intensely alive but had been taken too young – there was cancer, and two suicides. Having accepted those losses, I now found myself reliving the bereavements, and I saw that forgetting could be a protective mechanism. Daily life accumulates change in a gradual way, but the boxes of letters exploded into my consciousness, whirling me up into an atomic cloud of remembering. Together with the virus threat, the weeping, I wondered whether I was coming apart.

I had been writing a short story when the first lockdown came. I could not go on with it, but worse than not being able to write was not being able to read. Such a thing had never happened to me since I learned to read around the age of five. I picked up book after book, but my attention wandered after a few paragraphs. I would catch myself staring blankly at the page without having taken in a single word. Other writers described similar symptoms. I heard it was the fight-or-flight mechanism that kicks in when we are under threat: apparently, I was poised either to do battle or to flee, except that there was no visible enemy, and nowhere to run. It was a terrifying paralysis, and I had no idea when, or if, it might end.

Fortunately, the work of the previous year had just come to fruition with the publication of my novella *Murmurations*. I'd had to cancel the launch party, but when the book arrived it was its own reward – slender, with a beautiful cover, my deep pride in it became an anchor.

In the 1990s, when I lived on the Isle of Man, as I weeded my salt-wind-blown rose beds on clear days, I could see the Cumbrian coastline on the horizon. It was a view I hated, because it took in the nuclear reprocessing plant at Sellafield. But Seascale, the village close to the plant, was where John Ruskin loved to go to sketch dwarf roses and purple geraniums. And it was there, at Brantwood, that he created his unique garden.

Ruskin bought Brantwood when he was fifty-two, after the death of his parents, and arrived to take possession with a retinue of twelve gardeners. With their help he created winding pathways, and a private walled garden deep in the heart of a wood. It was a wild, unconventional place, its nooks and crannies planted with the wildflower specimens Ruskin gathered during his walks.

The story of his garden's decline mirrors Ruskin's own. As he aged, struggling through mental breakdown, the network of paths he had created gradually became overgrown. When his finances dwindled, there was the loss of paid help. Yet some of his most lucid writing dates from this period, as he looked back over his life. In his autobiography *Praeterita* he writes, 'My described life has thus become more amusing than I expected to myself, as I summoned its long past scenes for present scrutiny.'

If Ruskin had his own boxes of letters, the past they disgorged, among other troubling events, would have included his unconsummated marriage to Effie Gray, which ended in a scandalous annulment. Perhaps men are better at skimming over what they whispered and what they screamed, better at assimilating the crowding evidence of who they are and who they have been.

I picture Ruskin at Brantwood as a very old man, surrounded by the encroaching woods but able to gaze with delight on a posy of wildflowers, still straining each dusk after the cry of the elusive corncrake. For even in its dishevelled decline, Ruskin's garden shored him up against complete collapse, as gardens throughout history have soothed so many wounded. And perhaps some special gardens even have the power to cast a protective mantle over those who tend them. Like the Chelsea Physic Garden, with its gardeners who left to fight in the First World War: miraculously, every single one of them returned.

Here in Adelaide, my grandfather survived the French battlefields of that war, though with physical injuries that would plague him all his life. Then there were the horrors seen and heard that he never spoke of, not least that on the ship coming home, his best friend had jumped overboard to his death: a groin injury had left him unable to father children, and he had not been able to face his fiancé. My grandfather's post-war life was never completely easy; even into his old age there were visits to the repatriation hospital when his wounded leg flared up. But if his mind healed it was mostly achieved by gardening. I think of him wandering through his garden in the Adelaide Hills in the early morning with a cup of tea, pointing out and naming flowers for his grandchildren.

In *The Well Gardened Mind*, Sue Stuart-Smith tells the story of her grandfather, who was a submariner in the First World War. During the Gallipoli campaign he was taken prisoner, and spent time in a series of brutal labour camps in Turkey. The last was a cement factory, from which he eventually escaped, but after the long journey home he was so severely malnourished that he was given only a few months to live. Key to eventually regaining his health was a year-long horticultural course that had been set up to rehabilitate ex-servicemen.

Stuart-Smith, a psychiatrist as well as a gardener, writes of the therapeutic effects of working with our hands in a protected space, of how gardening allows our inner and outer worlds 'to coexist free from the pressures of everyday life'. In a garden we are able to hear and process our own, sometimes turbulent, thoughts.

During those weeks last year after Easter, when normal life ground to a halt and, along with the fear of viral contamination, there was the spectre of financial catastrophe and social collapse, the garden remained blessedly unchanged. Birds still came to bathe, and to drink from the water bowls; ripened fruit still weighted the branches of the quince and apple trees. The community garden was another, more spacious, walled refuge. Some of its ancient fruit trees have stood for more than a century, tended by gardeners through two world wars, and countless other crises. For a while, after everything else had shut, I was able to take a friend there to sit and talk, each bringing a thermos of tea and a sandwich, but as the social restrictions increased, it, too, closed to everyone but the plot holders.

Only my own garden offered respite. Through the perfect autumn days, I retreated to the veranda with Charlotte Brontë's *Jane Eyre* and soon became immersed in its candlelit world of great houses, of horses and carriages, of Jane's solitary walks at dusk through the countryside around Thornfield. The book's darkness and drama suited my mood, but most of all I was relieved to be able to read again. *Jane Eyre* broke my paralysis, and when I had finished, I was able to push on with other books.

I have been drawn to the artists and writers who have lingered in the twilight and expressed its beauty through their art. The peculiar power of dusk is that whatever we see then is about to vanish. Henri Le Sidaner was sensitive to this evanescence: he painted gardens at twilight, tables set with the remains of a meal or a private celebration, surrounded by the empty chairs of diners who had moved out of the picture. These depopulated gardens, which at first appear charming, carry a subtle undertone of menace.

Le Sidaner was in his mid-fifties in France during the First World War; I do not know whether he was involved in the fighting, but I am guessing the war must have shaken his sense of permanence. For there is a wistfulness to these twilight scenes, as if the artist sees that this simple pleasure is already slipping from the real world into the realm of memory, or dream.

Samuel Palmer, in his beautiful etching *The Bellman,* shows the town watchman strolling along a village street as the sun sinks, 'to bless the doors from nightly harm'. Folded cattle huddle in the gathering gloom, and in the foreground a small group of people are seated around a table under an arbour. In Palmer's *The Homeward Star*, people gather around an outdoor table beside a lit shepherd's hut. There is a sense of the landscape sinking into evening, and of repose at the end of the day's labour. But although Palmer's pastoral scenes appear idyllic, they were conceived against a background of political and social unrest, and the peace at dusk in his Kentish villages reflects Palmer's longing for a rural life that had already passed. Like other artists of the Romantic age, Palmer, a disciple of William Blake, depicted the outside world as it was shaped by his psyche.

In Sappho's beautiful fragment, though, the peace is real. It reminds me of those long northern hemisphere twilights, the hurrying to do things before nightfall, with children roaming the garden, shrieking, and becoming wilder as darkness approaches. One senses the lambs, the goats, being shepherded towards the byre, as the older children hurry homeward from woods and fields. The arc of the day is complete, and Sappho's Evening Star promises comfort, and return.

When I had wrestled the boxes of letters into a kind of order, they showed me that my life had an arc, and its rapidly ascending curve was not unlike those charting viral infections that we were seeing on the nightly news. The early years had been one long, fevered, upward rush, an aspirational push involving agitated movement, change for change's sake, the relentless quest for adventure. Past the midpoint, there was still some restlessness, but the curve soon began to flatten into a more tranquil decline.

Ageing, for all its indignities, does have about it an ineffable sense of return. I feel it in my growing preference for simplicity, in the way that my interest in adventure and entertainment has been replaced by a deepening commitment to the inner life, and to the completion of creative projects. I recognised the same arc in my mother as she entered old, old age. She preferred the ordinary over the exotic, and could extract intense pleasure from the smallest events – the first flowering of daffodils she had planted, or a slice of home-made cake.

Many years ago I visited a hypnotherapist, and she recorded a meditation for me that began in an extraordinarily calming way. I still use it if I am struggling to sleep, and it begins by imagining that I am surrounded by darkness; it is a wonderfully warm and welcoming darkness, and far out in that darkness is one tiny pinprick of white light. I am to imagine that this is a star, a private star, waiting to welcome me.

As I relax into this meditation, I often think it would be the perfect approach to death.

One family story demonstrates death and return in the most vivid manner. It concerns my husband – a pragmatic man, not given to visions or hallucinations – and the astonishing transformation he witnessed in the moments following his mother's death. He had been sitting at her bedside for hours, listening to her laboured breathing. When he realised that there was no longer an out-breath, he stood up and leaned close, to be sure.

What he saw was his elderly mother in the process of being transformed into a young woman. He describes it as like a backwards ageing, a slow-motion film in which his mother grew younger and younger, until her face on the pillow was the face of the young woman he had known as a small child. All the lines were erased; even her hair turned from ash grey to blonde. After a stunned minute, in which he stood frozen, he went to call a nurse. By the time he returned to the room, his mother once more looked her age. Through the years we have puzzled over this strange experience, but have never come to any conclusion.

My hope for the end of life is that it will be like stepping into a Samuel Palmer etching – calmness at day's end, though without the background unrest. Then again, an ideal death might feel like entering Sappho's poem, less an ending than a return. I like to imagine a scented dusk in which a blackbird sings, while the scattered self is gathered back to Mother Earth.

Sheet lightning flickers, and all the neighbourhood dogs are barking; it's not yet dark, but the birds have stopped flying. Before the streetlight comes on, I try to photograph the garden. The pillar roses are exquisite just now, but a wrecking rain is on the way. Always, this happens. It's as if their beauty magnetises some great universal anger or despoiling force.

Every minute of the downpour is torture. The Pierre de Ronsard roses will be waterlogged, while the more delicate roses will be dashed to the ground. In between downpours, I rush out to shake water from the many-pleated blooms of the pillar roses.

Afterwards, in the calm, everything is damp and limp with something about it of the aftermath of sex. The garden is curiously silent. More silent than before, as if the thunder established some new norm of noise. Away over the hills I still hear the odd low rumble. There is trouble in foreign parts.

I move from bush to bush, shaking water from the roses.

Extract from my garden journal, November 2021

Chapter 19

Life After Life

I have never found a set of spiritual beliefs that unravelled life's meaning for me, or provided lasting consolation. Time and again, some calamity or other has forced the question: how can there be a God if this can happen, and this? Yet there have been rare moments when meaning seemed almost within reach – falling in love, marriage, the arrival of a child, even publishing a book one has thrown one's whole self into. Possibly I have mistaken happiness for meaning. Yet even the most luminous happiness seems to be by nature fleeting, whereas I would expect meaning to endure.

My grasp of science is shaky, and I have never dared to write poetry, but if there is a meaning to life that a human mind can grasp, I'm guessing it lies in a fusion of poetry with physics, and even astronomy – spheres of knowledge that the American astrophysicist Carl Sagan famously explored. Sagan said that science is, at least in part, 'informed worship', and what could be more worthy of worship than our blue planet with its cargo of souls, spinning in space – perhaps alone, perhaps as yet simply undiscovered, or unvisited – supposing there is anyone out there to make a visit.

Being born, living, growing old and dying, as far as we understand these states of being, all occur within our vexed relationship with time. Time in space is measured in light years, and the great mystery is that this light reaches us across an unimaginable distance, and travels away to an equally unimaginable, unknowable destination.

I am not convinced of Christianity's Heaven, or its Hell; I don't know whether we will be reborn, as some religions believe. But whenever I try to conjure an image of life after this earthly life, if there is to be such a thing, it is a place where time is light, and where time, overtaking and enfolding us, fills us with its radiance.

There is a long moment just on nightfall when the garden is at its most seductive. New shapes emerge; it is a place of hurried, half-seen flitterings, this evening hour that is older even than the word 'vespers'. Weather and season shape each slow dissolving, at times conjuring moths, mosquitoes, scents of compost and leaf mould, or the rare blue-strobe flicker of sheet lightning beyond the hills. Wings beat unseen towards distant treetops, and time's linearity – implacable in sunlight – becomes as mutable as thought, as dream.

The blue hour is the first and most bewitching of the dimming evening's stages. Known as civil twilight, this threshold arrives when the sun dips below the horizon by up to six degrees, when the first faint stars are visible. Pale flowers float as shadows deepen, and white objects rush to meet the eye. In spring and summer dusks, when crickets creak, and the blackbird pours out his last …

thrilling solo, I would, if I could, capture and hold the garden in this moment of ecstatic sinking. I am never without my camera then; I write, but the blue hour is elusive.

Nautical twilight is reached when the sun dips below the horizon by between six and twelve degrees. Both horizon and stars are visible, a boon to navigating sailors. The third and last of evening's stages is astronomical twilight, which arrives when the sun dips to eighteen degrees below the horizon. The sinking of the day is complete when the last shimmer of sunlight disperses. Nightfall arrives then, as it must, though in truth, night in the garden does not fall, but rises inexorably from the roots and soil and shadowy under-planting; night swallows the deepest colours first.

Extract from my garden journal, November 2021

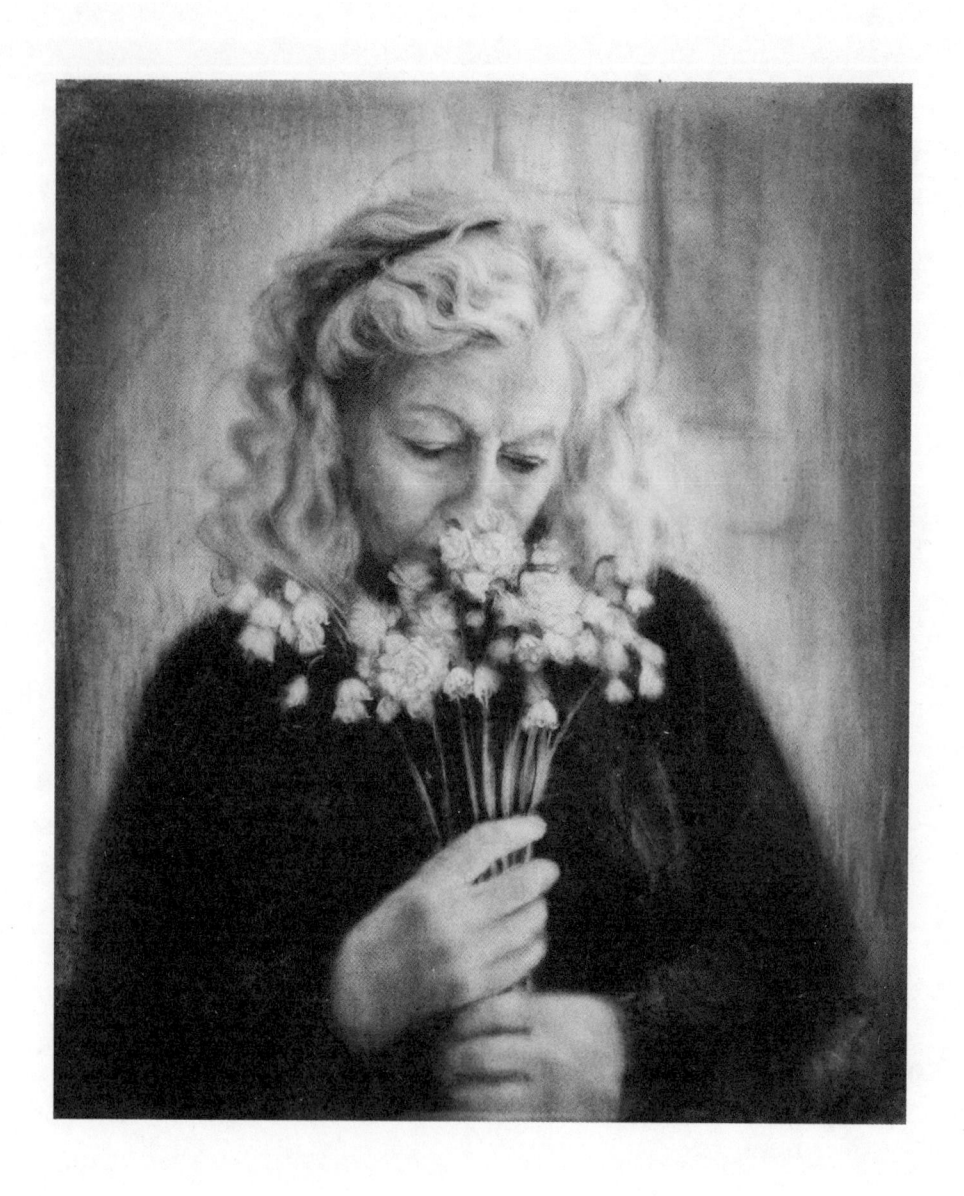

Chapter 20

Okay, Bloomer

> Do you have the patience to wait
> till your mud settles and the water is clear?
> *Tao Te Ching*, Lao Tzu

The Vietnamese monk Thich Nhat Hanh likens human suffering to mud, and reminds us that mud is needed in order for a lotus to grow. 'The mud doesn't smell so good, but the lotus flower smells very good. If you don't have mud, the lotus won't manifest. You can't grow lotus flowers on marble. Without mud, there can be no lotus.' By seventy, most of us have waded through plenty of mud. But this is the time when the mud finally settles and the lotus can bloom. At seventy, it's now or never.

In her book *The Long Life*, Helen Small, professor of English Language and Literature at Merton College, Oxford, asks, 'At what point in a life can we measure its happiness?' In the United Kingdom, a survey of more than 300,000 adults found that happiness peaks between the ages of sixty-five and seventy-nine, while the forty-five to fifty-nine category records the lowest levels of life satisfaction and the highest levels of anxiety. In the stages of ageing, adults between sixty-five and eighty-four are known as the Young Old; it is a life period identified as the 'third age', following on from the 'first age' (childhood) and the 'second age' (parenting). For most of us in the third age, though not all, our working lives are behind us, which may be one of the reasons this stage is said to be the golden age of adulthood.

The generation known as Baby Boomers are now firmly within this Young Old age range; some of us have been there for a while. But Boomers have the potential to become Bloomers, capable of doing ageing well. By that I don't mean achieving the kind of airbrushed reality displayed on hoardings outside retirement villages, the 'positive ageing' model pumped out by those with an interest in profiting from retirees. That is a model that sets up the possibility of failure. I mean what if we were to simply reject the beliefs about ageing with which we've been primed and embrace a sense of ongoingness, of moving always towards the next adventure?

The French philosopher Henri Bergson conceived of an enduring life force (*élan vital*) that progresses and is continually developing. For Bergson, life is a dynamic process in which the material present, the actual moment, is suffused with the virtuality of memory. Lived time (*la durée*) is not the time of calendars and clocks but of the inner life, and whether *la durée* seems to pass quickly or slowly is influenced by our subjective memories, and by our anticipation of the future. 'Certainly, pure consciousness does not perceive time as a sum of units of duration: left to itself, it has no means and even no reason to measure time.'

Bergson praised the insight of those who shake off the views embedded by social conditioning:

Fortunately, some are born with spiritual immune systems that sooner or later give rejection to the illusory world view grafted upon them from birth through social conditioning. They begin sensing that something is amiss, and start looking for answers ... Each step of the journey is made by following the heart instead of following the crowd, and by choosing knowledge over the veils of ignorance.

Age can bring serious challenges, as I've discovered in this landmark year. And while I have been fortunate to receive an early diagnosis and treatment, I realise this may not be the end of things. As the naturopath explained after I'd recovered from surgery: 'Your body has made a cancer, and the important thing now is to avoid the conditions that allowed that to happen.' I try to trust in the process of follow-up monitoring laid out by the health professionals looking after me and, as much as I am able to, I stick to the naturopathic advice on diet and exercise, although that tin of sardines in the pantry remains unopened. I have resisted searching the internet for outcomes and advice, knowing it will only stoke my anxiety. Because I'd be lying if I said I am not anxious.

Cancer changes you. As with any trauma, the life you lead afterwards is not the same as before. In some ways it's better. I am less inclined now to hold on to things that serve no good purpose; I feel in my whole body the preciousness of the people and things I love, and also the fleeting nature of our time together. I know that I am lucky to be alive, as does every old person I've spoken to. And although the time ahead is shorter than it once was, shorter than most of us would like, we are not people at the end of things but people still on our way, for, to quote Henri Bergson: 'To exist is to change, to change is to mature, to mature is to go on creating oneself endlessly.'

~

It is late November, and my garden has hit an ecstatic high note of beauty and wildness. Among plants I've nurtured for more than a decade are others that have drifted in on the wind, and even a few specimens that belonged to an earlier gardener have reappeared after an extended dormancy. Inevitably, there are weeds, but I look past them to the Christmas lilies, given to me by my mother. They are six feet tall and already releasing a heady scent that envelops me as I step through the gate from the street.

I stand and breathe it in, and there is a rush of joy for the ongoingness of my mother's gifts to me – not only of these lilies but of my own life, and that of my brother. There is a twinge of sadness, too, that she is not here to see how her lilies have outdone themselves this spring. But when she brought them to me as bulbs she must have known they would return year after year, stirring memory, giving pleasure. If I were to leave this house for another, of all the plants in the garden that are in some way special, it would be those lilies I would dig up and take with me.

The roses are also flowering madly in a second flush of loveliness, and the self-seeded Queen Anne's lace – one of the garden's wildest elements – fills every gap with its snowy, snowflake-like umbels. It even springs up in cracks in the paving, somewhat like the stray thoughts that flit through my mind when I'm out walking, or when I'm supposed to be asleep. In the language of flowers, Queen Anne's lace represents sanctuary, and to return to the garden is always to gratefully re-enter a private and consoling space where the outside world can be held at bay.

The American garden writer Elizabeth Lawrence famously insisted that 'There is a garden in every childhood, an enchanted place, where colours are brighter, the air is softer, and the morning more fragrant than ever again'. But I would argue that there should be a garden in every old age, that age itself is a garden – an enchanted place, where colours veer towards those only visible to birds, colours that for a lifetime have eluded our human vision. In the garden of age, every in-breath is taken with gratitude for the availability of air, and each morning is more fragrant than the one before.

Given that a garden is always a reflection of the gardener, matching the season of spring with age may seem counter-intuitive. But spring's abundance, its flowery abandon, feels exactly right for this life stage when the past is brimful, the present is intense, and the future is fated to unfold in a kaleidoscopic shift of influences. Although I am only at the start of Young Old Age, already it feels like a place where one's eccentricities can mingle unchecked with the tamer elements of everyday life – just like my own garden, in fact, where weeds intermingle with roses and lilies. Even my run-in this year with cancer does not incline me to identify with another season. If anything, a cancer diagnosis intensifies the present; it heightens the delight of being alive and having come through; it holds out the promise of a second spring.

But the spring garden's high-pitched beauty is ephemeral. Everything in it is always moving *from* something *towards* something else. On this particular day the slender stems of the Queen Anne's lace stand motionless, as if awaiting the Bureau of Meteorology's predicted storm. Heavy rain, when it comes, will pummel the great cream trumpets of the lilies; it will waterlog the roses. The brush fence, and the cordon of fruit trees around the perimeter – quince, pear, plum – offer some protection from strong winds, but it will not be enough.

The only thing to do during this lull before the weather breaks is to give the garden one's full attention. So I stand before the lilies, noticing how gracefully they intermingle with the Queen Anne's lace, how serenely all the white notes sing together. I pick roses to bring indoors; I take photographs, and even do a little video sweep around the whole of the garden. Tellingly, the birds are silent. On most days the shrubs are a-rustle with the dart and flutter of sparrows and honeyeaters, while mudlarks and spotted doves visit the drinking bowls and bird bath. Eventually I spy a lone blackbird perched pensively on our neighbours' chimney, and I can tell that, like the rest of his feathered fellows, he senses the onslaught of wind and rain that is slowly sweeping towards us from the west.

While the garden exists at this peak of perfection I bring as much intensity as I can muster to inhabiting and absorbing its beauty. *Love hard in the present moment*, sing the lilies; *see as if tomorrow you will be blind*, hums the Queen Anne's lace. I do my best to obey, and to not diminish the joy of the present abundance by anticipating its imminent destruction.

~

Those of us who have lived most of our lives in the 20th century are often portrayed as inept with technology, when in fact most of us own and use smart phones, tablets and smart watches, and have adapted to email and the internet. We are the first generation to use technology to benefit our ageing. And if, as Henry Ford insisted, you are only old when you stop learning, and that anyone who keeps learning stays young, then with online classes and YouTube tutorials it has never been easier to stay young: to learn something new or join an online class, or download an app and work on your fitness in private and at your own pace.

Undertaking anything new can provide a sense of purpose and structure; it can prove to us that we are not too old to learn, to become fitter or to embark on some interesting adventure. If you need inspiration, an online search will turn up many older people with amazing achievements. For example, in the United States, cancer survivor Harriette Thompson ran her first marathon in 1999 to support friends who were ill with leukaemia. Harriette was seventy-six. Since then she has broken records, including being the oldest woman ever to run a marathon, and to run a half-marathon. Harriette was ninety-one when she completed the San Diego marathon (for the fifteenth time) in 7 hours, 7 minutes and 42 seconds.

At seventy-nine, Wang Deshun became a catwalk model and instant internet sensation during Fashion Week in Beijing. When asked in an interview with *GQ* magazine about how he kept in shape and maintained the youthful, mesmerising grace that would be the envy of decades-younger men, Wang said simply, 'I pursue nowness. That's what I do.'

Having been a factory worker, an actor and theatre director, and somehow surviving China's Cultural Revolution, Wang first stepped into a gym at fifty, and at fifty-seven he returned to the stage, creating an extraordinary form of pantomime art he called 'Living Sculptures'. At seventy he redoubled his efforts in the gym, and on the cusp of eighty, after his catwalk performance, he was dubbed 'The Hottest Grandpa'.

Wang says, 'I still have some dreams to explore. Believe me, potential can be explored. When you think it's too late, be careful you don't let that become your excuse for giving up. No one can keep you from success except yourself.'

In 2003, at the age of seventy, Japanese climber Yūichirō Miura became the oldest person to reach the summit of Mount Everest. Miura had heart surgery in 2006 and 2007, but in May 2013, at the age of eighty, he again became the oldest person to reach the summit. It was his third time at the top of the world's tallest mountain, and he revealed that he would like to try again at ninety.

By October 2008, Japanese sailor Minoru Saitō had already accomplished a record-breaking seven solo journeys around the world, but now he planned to travel west to east, a famously challenging route that works against prevailing winds and currents. After an epic 1080-day journey, Saitō returned home. At seventy-seven, he became the world's oldest person to sail around the world, and the oldest to do it the 'wrong way'.

'I feel very young in both mind and body, and I feel I'm in great shape,' Saitō said. 'I'm already thinking about my next trip. I'd like to head to Greenland and Alaska.'

Closer to home, much-loved Australian artist Grace Cossington Smith began work on her painting *Interior in Yellow* in 1962, at the age of seventy. Before she could finish it, she fell and broke her hip while living alone in Turramurra. Over the next two years she went on to complete the painting and, despite her outward appearance of frailty, *Interior in Yellow* speaks of an inner strength and resilience and dazzles with its vibrant colour. Her last painting, *Still life with white cup and saucer*, finished a decade later, shows the deep pleasure Cossington Smith found in everyday objects.

At 109, Eileen Kramer is Australia's oldest dancer and choreographer. In 2014, to mark her hundredth birthday, she crowdfunded, choreographed and performed a dance piece called *The Early Ones*. In 2019, she entered a self-portrait for the Archibald Prize, becoming the award's oldest ever contributor. Asked where her energy comes from, and whether there's a secret to dancing into old age, Kramer said that she banishes the words 'old' and 'age' from her vocabulary.

'I say: I'm not old, I've just been here a long time and learnt a few things along the way. I don't feel how people say you should feel when you're old. My attitude to creating things is identical to when I was a child.'

On a much reduced scale, my own activities at this age give me pleasure. Anyone who has maintained a skill over many years will have at last emerged from their apprenticeship. We can expect our practice to have become almost effortless. I hope to write for as long as I can still hold a pen, and with luck and a fair wind I will continue to be published. I read widely, and take part in literary events both in my own small circle and in Australia's wider literary culture. Then there is family life, the house and the garden. I could never have managed all of this as a young woman. I simply didn't have the confidence or the experience for the writing, although it was a dream I secretly cherished. And, though I always felt gratitude for the roof over my head, and the garden, if I had one, those were the years when I was running to keep up, striving to get somewhere, although where that might have been I was never certain. With the slower pace of this age, the mud whose murk so often clouded my thinking in those younger years has finally begun to settle.

If wisdom has been gleaned in this year of paying close attention to ageing, it has often come from conversations with people who generously shared their thoughts and experiences of where life has taken them at seventy, or eighty, and beyond. I found more courage, more humour, more happiness than might be expected, despite the obvious challenges. On encountering lives that have been shaped by every force imaginable, from the British Empire to family struggles and instances of serendipity, I realised that age is something to be honoured and accepted. And just occasionally I've been left with a sense that one might find ways to exist outside of time, or to simply refuse to age at all.

I am sustained by the thought that this is always where life was leading, this vantage point with the longest view, where we can be more ourselves than we have ever been. Perhaps this is what Shakespeare meant when he wrote, 'The golden age is before us, not behind us.' Indeed, the years between sixty-nine and eighty-four have long been referred to as golden years. Beyond seventy, we are short of time, and we know it. But there are unexpected joys, too – small ecstasies, really – that I for one would not have understood, or even noticed, when I was younger. Now my aim each day is to live with heightened awareness, to breathe deep the joy of being alive – to literally smell the roses. I want to read more, write more, listen to more music; I want to love those I love with full attention; I want to forgive, and forget, and remember; I want to be more generous, with myself as well as with others. I want to own less, and think more.

Above all, I want to be intensely present.

The American psychologist and author Mary Pipher notes that 'old age, especially in the last hard years, is really a search for a place in the universe. The old look for their existential place. They ask, "How did my life matter?" "Was my time well spent?" "What did I mean to others?"' Far from being a cut-off point, threescore years and ten is an age at which the shape and pattern of one's life may finally be understood. There, with a rich experience to draw on, and a stretch of precious time ahead, we might, if we are so inclined, apply our hearts to wisdom.

By a stroke of serendipity, I am putting the finishing touches to this final piece on the last day of December in a year that began in devastating fashion with my mother's death. Still mourning her loss, I weathered a diagnosis of cancer and survived a major surgery. In between times, I spent many hours talking to old people. I read many books and planted and harvested flowers, herbs and fruit. I recorded the slow march of the seasons as they passed through this small plot of land, and realised again that garden time is not 'clock time', that its rhythms are more nourishing and that, as with gardens, age itself is made more pleasurable by elements of wildness. By that I mean that reaching a stage of life where one is no longer bound by the expectations and opinions of others is freeing, so that if the crone in me decides to grow grey hair to my waist, no one can stop me. Or if I choose never again to cook meat and dine instead on chopped beetroot and baby spinach leaves, no one can persuade me against it. This freedom to be one's true self is old age's gift.

Standing in the garden at dusk remains one of my deepest pleasures. I look around and know how fortunate I am to be alive in this strange and beautiful cosmos. It is easy then to be not just *in* the garden, but *of* the garden, part of the fabric of the natural world in which one is held by the motions and influences of the planets, by the turning and returning seasons, held by unnameable forces one can only guess at. Some evenings, fruit bats pass overhead, indistinct and mysterious in the grainy light. At other times, crickets sing or a slender new moon gleams above the rooftops. I float free then, somewhere outside of time, in memory lush with past springs, golden summers and autumns, the bulbs of all my winters, of all the precious seasons still to come. My body may be old, but the self inside is ageless. I say to myself: Okay, Bloomer, the Golden Age is now. Now is the time to flower.

Appendices

Appendices

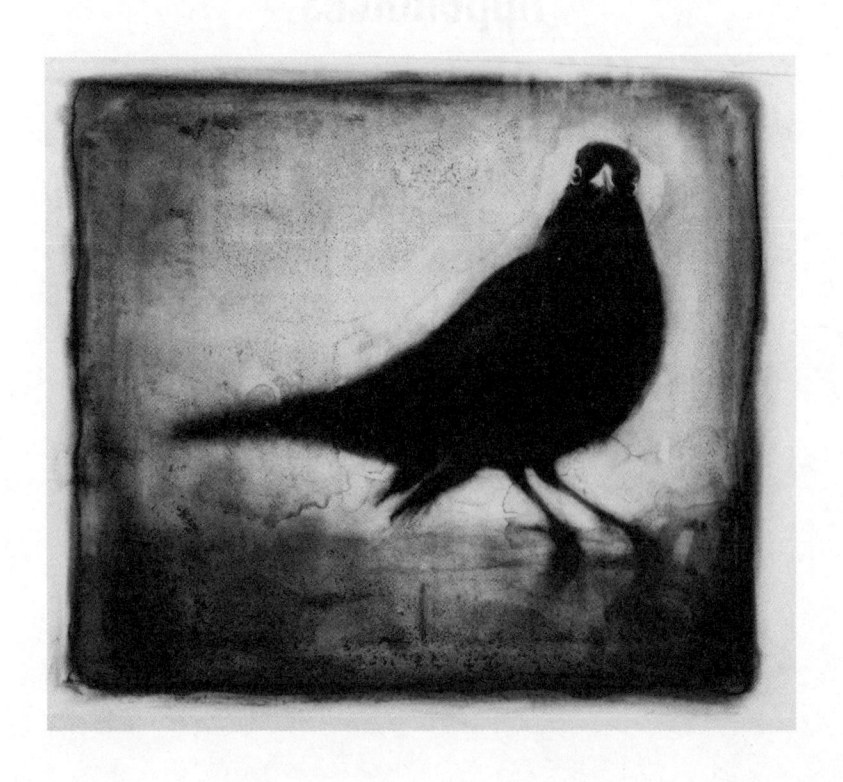

We Need to Talk About Ageing

Questioning the purpose of old age began as a private, reflective process. But before long I was exploring the formidable forces at work in the universe – the mysteries of time and memory, birth and death, and the possibility (or not) of the existence of something either side of those momentous bookends. My thinking and reading took place against a background hum of old-age-as-decline, the pedal tone of our society's ageism. From libraries, and often from their storage facilities, I unearthed books by bygone thinkers who had pondered the same problems: poets and philosophers, novelists, Nobel Prize winners, whose words have slipped from sight because for a long time we have not wanted to think or talk about growing old.

Eventually I sought out other old people, to tap in to their experiences of ageing. Many convivial hours of conversation ensued, over coffee or tea, sometimes with cake, and I saw that within each of them – as within me – lay multitudes of younger selves, laid down layer upon layer, each steeped in the music of its time, each a rich repository of memories. Some people were doing well, some not so well. We discussed the hard parts of our lives as well as the good parts, and occasionally one or both of us shed a few tears. What we were all agreed on is that we are living in a time and place in which old people are not valued, and that ageism is damaging – not just to old people, but to younger people who could benefit from better role models for their own ageing.

I began to wonder how we could bring about social change, or at the very least a change of tone around the topic of ageing. It seemed an insurmountable task. And then, at a writing festival, I heard Dr Michael Mohammed Ahmad, founding director of Sweatshop, a literacy movement in Western Sydney, passionately declare that marginalised people can only instigate change by kickstarting it from within the group itself. I shot up straight in my chair, electrified by this truth. Old people exist largely in the margins, but unlike other socially diminished groups they have been shuffled there by those who will one day share the same experience. I thought of other marginalised voices that have been raised in protest – Black voices, queer voices, trans voices, female voices, from suffragettes to the #MeToo movement.

Ageism's negative impact on the health and wellbeing of older people is well documented, yet ageism is so deeply embedded in our culture that its surface signs – jokey greeting cards, 'anti-ageing' products in the beauty industry – are widely thought acceptable. How have we allowed this to happen? We've allowed it by not thinking or talking about ageing or ageism. Instead we've let ourselves be brainwashed into believing that ageing is somehow shameful, it's distasteful and ugly, ageing is something to be feared and fought against and denied, to be pushed from sight, despite the fact that it's happening to every one of us every day of the week. Because the passage of time affects all things, from the greenfly on the roses to kings and queens on their thrones. Even stones age, their surfaces weathered smooth by unimaginable quantities of time.

As a generation shaped during the social revolution of the sixties, its protest movements and its music, Boomers could and should be doing something about changing the ageing narrative. Instead of being age denialists, we need to talk about the challenges and rewards of ageing – to everyone, from our own families to neighbours, local community groups, social media contacts, our GPs and our members of parliament. Ageing is a natural process, and old age, for those lucky enough to reach it, is the culmination of a life. Perhaps, if we only stopped to reflect, it might even contain life's meaning. In accepting this, we need to rescue the word 'old' from its position as an insult, and reclaim it, using it as a term of respect. Old people need a flag, a logo, they need their voices to be heard. Because every part of a life is precious, and old lives *do* matter. Change *can* happen one conversation at a time.

These extracts from some of the conversations I've had are a window into the thoughts, ideas and experiences of people doing ageing with fortitude and grace. Some of them may be a little further along on the path we ourselves must follow. But if we were hiking a perilous mountain trail, wouldn't we listen to what those ahead of us had seen and heard and know?

Philippa: eighty
On surviving a serious stroke and moving into aged care

CL: It's good to see you. Are you in reasonable health now?

P: Yes, well, not long after I came here, I remember it was like a switch being thrown. I'd think: I remember that, and I remember that. And all my memory came back, and then slowly I felt as if I was healing. But when I first came here, on my notes from the hospital they said I had dementia, and for a while I was somebody else. It's what I call now my 'false memory', and I know a lot of it's not true, but I remember it as if it is. I don't know whether it was a dream, or I was in a coma, but I remember being part of a militant Chinese army for women. It's so real to me, that we were fighting for something, a guerrilla group fighting another group. So I had another persona for a while.

CL: Perhaps what you're remembering is some kind of internal struggle to survive after your stroke, and the surgery.

P: Yes. And the other thing is, I knew that I was in hospital, and I know where it really is, but in my head it was by the sea. I sent my son a note once asking him to come and pick me up, and I said I was waiting at the Grange railway station. I know that's not true, but for a time my brain was living another life.

The place I was living in was like a boarding house, an old, grand boarding house with timber frame windows, and we were near a golf course. There were people that I met there, and it was by the sea. And although they said I was in hospital, in my head I was somewhere else.

CL: Did you tell the medical people about the boarding house and the army?

P: Well, I did, and they didn't take a lot of notice. It's what I call my false memory, and I think that's important. Because they talk about people having false memories about things.

CL: Was it like any place you've ever been to in real life? Was it coming up from the past, or was it entirely new?

P: It was entirely new. I think it must have been when I was having my operation, because I remember I got off the train, it must have been Grange, and I was saying, 'I've got nowhere to live, I've got nowhere to sleep tonight, where am I going to stay?' And I came across somebody that I didn't really know, and they said, 'Oh, I go down to this place here. They'll let you stay the night.' So I went down to this place, which was really Flinders Hospital, and then this guy said, 'I stay here, you stay with me and I'll get you a room.' And I stayed in this place, and the lady said, 'Yes, you can stay tonight, and you can probably stay tomorrow night, too.' It didn't look like a hospital, it looked like a grand old boarding house. Perhaps that's when I was under anaesthetic, I don't know.

CL: Amazing!

P: After I'd been here a while in respite care, they sent up a specialist, who interviewed me, and then said, 'You're fine. We don't think we need to see you anymore.'

CL: What does your typical day look like? Do you have a routine?

P: I've got to the stage now where I can get myself out of bed, and shower. I make my bed and tidy my room. And, of course, there's structure with meals. I say to myself, 'Gee, I'm glad I don't do the washing up anymore!'

CL: Covid has changed a lot of things for all of us, and you would have been here during the lockdown.

P: I arrived just at the beginning of the lockdown. And it has, it's changed how we interact with people. Understandably, with so many rules about Covid, people stopped coming; it sort of became too hard to do. A lot of us did feel very isolated.

CL: But it's eased up a bit now, and so you get out? Do you see people?

P: I don't see people as much, and I think that happens in every case. After a while people stop coming, or they get on with their lives. It's a bit hard when you're isolated here, but it's the reality of life.

CL: Was there a point at which you began to feel old?

P: I suppose moving here brought that home to me. You've got to sell the house and give away all your belongings. I was lucky, and the kids did most of that for me. They got Vinnies to take the furniture. But on a couple of days I went to the house, and I thought, well, I don't really know what I want to take with me. What can you take and put in one room? You can't fit a whole lifetime into one room. I just had to say to myself, 'I can't think about it. It's got to be done, and if I think about it, I won't be able to move forward.' And then I had a moment where I thought that if the place burned down and there was nothing left, I couldn't do anything about that either. So it's much the same thing, isn't it? Your life just disappears. You have to take a deep breath and say, okay, that's the way it is. Because otherwise you can't move forward.

Jo: eighty-three
On mindful eating, diet, exercise and refusing the label 'old'

CL: I've heard you refer to your 'beautiful simple life'. I know you live very quietly.

J: To the extent that I really only talk to S [a friend] on the phone, and I haven't spoken to her for about a week.

CL: Do you like it that way?

J: I enjoy it that way. Thinking back to a starting point of the idea of ageing as a concept, I wanted every day of my life to be mine. The actual concept of growing old in the sense of pensions, superannuation – the whole concept of that stretching ahead as an idea of life – was like a nightmare to me. I couldn't imagine living a life on those terms. And the actual idea, the labels – pensions, superannuation – the idea of looking at people going off every day in their suits, I thought: what's the point of a life like that? So that's why I decided to work extremely hard, which I did, inventing things, working on houses, working on cars, everything to get this financial independence where we owned our own house. So that's what I did. I achieved that.

CL: How long did that take?

J: I effectively retired from the normal workforce on my thirty-fourth birthday.

CL: That's a huge achievement.

J: I gave up engineering, and people in that area I was working in, inventing things for, when I said I was going to become an artist now, they said: 'Art? What's this art business? Jo, you've got this list of patents.' I had patents dotted around the world in my name. That was a starting point. Anyway, I need to show you something. [We go into another room, where Jo points out a black-and-white photograph, blown up, on the wall. It shows a young boy in a garden wearing a white shirt and dark shorts, and his whole figure seems to emanate a feeling of liveliness and joy.]

That was me at three and a half. I relate to that as an idea, as a concept of my life. I want to maintain that freshness, that childlike freshness. You've got no responsibilities; every day is a new day. You're looking at things in a different light, you're aware of everything around you. That's what I wanted to maintain, that feeling through my life – I'm talking age-wise. My concept of my ageing is there [in the childhood photograph].

CL: That's wonderful!

J: I've always held that, and I've maintained that, so that was my decision of giving up work, I wanted to be independent, I wanted every day to be My Day. Hence no television, no media, being cut off – no telephone, only outside telephone calls, no mobile phone, no computer. Just shutting off all those things, but every day is an important day to me. I'm trying to get age in perspective, and that is the starting point, maintaining that freshness in my life.

CL: It's a unique perspective, Jo, which is what I expected. It's the reason I wanted to talk to you about this.

J: So that's the starting point. Hence the very limited people that I talk to. That's evolved over the years, leading into a very quiet, meditative, separate life from people, shutting off from people, and also not having an association with old people, elderly people, who have an attitude to life that's not mine. So it's important that I don't associate with people with that sort of attitude. Thinking of life and death on those terms, of ageing and feeling old. And you look at people and they're *feeling* old, and they talk about *being* old.

CL: You think age is a state of mind that is best avoided?

J: That's right. It's about maintaining that freshness, and valuing each day for what it is, as an amazing experience. We experience an amazing physical life. I want to maintain that feeling every day, hence the isolation from media and all these sorts of things that just load your mind, and also load your mind conditionally, relative to age. The whole presentation of our society is relative to age.

CL: There's no value placed on age.

J: Every approach to age in our society is completely wrong. But on top of that you've got the idea of people dying, and people being afraid of age, and the concept of funerals. I never go to funerals, it's all wrong. The idea of funerals is wrong, for me. In my will, I've laid out that there should be no normal ceremony, it should be an exciting event. Literally, there should be a party celebrating my new adventure. I'm setting out on a new adventure. It's a new experience.

CL: What does your normal day look like? Do you have a routine?

J: When I wake up I do fifty sit-ups. I then go to my exercise bike and I do three kilometres. The first kilometre is a warm-up, the next is fairly hard work, and the final one is absolutely flat out. So that's the start of the day. And then I have two slices of bread for breakfast. No jam, no sweeteners, just plain bread with Flora margarine on it to get some fat in my system. I don't eat anything during the day, and then at 6.15 I eat 400 to 450 grams of bananas. Ripe bananas, bags of ripe bananas. So 400 grams, and then vegetables. I drink half a litre of soy milk every day, and am basically conscious of food and getting lots of protein. Controlled fat, very controlled sugar, and just basic, essential eating every day. So that's my pattern, and then I go for a walk in the morning, about a half-an-hour walk, and every afternoon I ride out in different directions. These are my afternoon rides, when it's not too cold. It's getting a little bit cold now, and I've got no insulation, being as thin as I am.

CL: Tell me about the bananas. Why that quantity, and why are they so good for you?

J: Well, bananas, if you look at the nutrition books, they've got more nutritious goodies in them than all other fruit. They're easy to digest. And they're just very sensible things to eat.

CL: They're almost a complete food, aren't they?

J: They're a very basic food, so a nice healthy thing. I've been eating 400 grams for years now. And they need to be ripe ones. I can't eat hard bananas.

CL: You must have to shop for them quite often to have them fresh and ripe.

J: Sometimes shops put aside ripe bananas, because as soon as they get little marks on them people won't buy them. I've been buying bags of bananas for a dollar, which I keep for several days, or a week. I've got trays of bananas. You wouldn't believe my fridge. [We go and look in the fridge, which is indeed quite full of bananas, as well as neat containers of vegetables.] And they become sweeter as they get riper, of course.

CL: How do you eat them?

J: I spend about a quarter of an hour eating a banana. I peel the skin back and use a knife to take slices off the top, slice by slice. I eat it very carefully and enjoy each mouthful rather than taking a big bite. I eat very slowly and very carefully, and I enjoy each mouthful.

CL: It's a mindful process – what is now termed mindfulness. You've been practising this for years, but it's a kind of buzzword in the present.

J: Yes, and the idea of it. I mean, I love the idea of eating, the actual concept of eating, so I enjoy every mouthful as part of the ritual of actually eating and experiencing the process of eating. I mean, we're talking about ageing, and an attitude to life, which is all part of the whole thing, of course, an attitude, to everything. It encompasses the whole idea of ageing, and of how you feel, age-wise.

Florence: eighty-one
On migration, road rage, surviving domestic violence, and a passion for playing bridge

CL: Can I start by asking your age at your last birthday?

F: Eighty-one.

CL: You look radiant.

F: Oh, darling, thank you. I thank God for makeup and hair. I don't think they even know how old I am at bridge, because when they ask, I say, 'Oh well, I'm twenty-five and a few months.'

CL: Have you always lived in Australia?

F: No, I was born in India. My father was in the British Army stationed in India while India was under British rule. We got run out when there was Partition, and he decided to go to Pakistan. He had a home in England, and my sister and I were put into boarding school in Pakistan, and my brothers were in boarding school in England. Then [my parents] spent half of the year in England when the boys were on holiday, and half in Pakistan.

When my sister was eighteen and I was seventeen, we came to Australia because my mum's family were all here. We came straight from a convent, had never done anything or been anywhere, and my grandmother, who we were coming to live with, was so excited – because she hadn't seen us since we were two and three – that she had a heart attack and finished up in the hospital.

My grandmother's house was one of those little cottages, and we thought it was the absolute pits because we came from what we thought was a mansion, but everybody we knew [in Pakistan] had a house like that. It took us probably an hour to find the toilet because it was outside. We had no idea – we'd never cooked, because we'd had servants, never had to wash or iron anything. We'd never even seen a kitchen.

My grandmother's got the fridge full of food, but we wouldn't have recognised a chop from a steak. The neighbour came in to say, 'Welcome to Australia, sorry about your grandma, and can we do anything for you?' We were very shy, but we got up enough courage to ask could they light the stove so we could maybe cook something. The neighbour turned the stove on for us. We thought the best thing we could do, the only thing we recognised, we could make an egg sandwich. So we put four eggs in a saucepan and put it on the stove, and we turned the TV on because we hadn't seen television since we were in England. After about half an hour the eggs exploded, because we hadn't put any water in the saucepan. We spent our first night in Australia cleaning my grandmother's kitchen, then we made jam and bread and cried our eyes out because we didn't want to be here.

CL: Tell me about how you went from making a jam sandwich, and exploding eggs, to learning how things worked. What was the next day like?

F: I think it was the neighbour who realised how useless we were and rang one of the family and said these girls are going to starve to death if you don't rescue them. My uncle came, and they decided they'd better take us to their place. We were so flabbergasted to think that our servants [in Pakistan] lived in better quarters, at least as far as I was concerned.

CL: Modern life seems faster, doesn't it?

F: There's so much road rage. Not long ago, as I was turning left, I cut this fellow off. His face was red, and he was obviously swearing. I stopped at the next lights and he stopped behind me, and I thought, he's going to kill me. He got out of the car and started walking towards me, and I got out of the car, and before he could say anything – I could see he was absolutely livid – I said to him, 'Oh my God, I'm so sorry that I cut you off! I really didn't see you, and thank God you're a good driver otherwise you would have hit me.' And he just stopped in his tracks. And he said, 'Oh, all right, then.' And he turned around and got into his car.

CL: The key was that you told him he was such a good driver! I'm going to keep that up my sleeve next time I need to disarm an angry road-rage person.

F: I think I dodged a bullet. To be honest, I was frightened.

CL: Do you think much about the past? It's the past, and memory, that seems to hold us in place.

F: One of the partners I play with at bridge has dementia. But he's such a lovely man, and I know he so looks forward to coming to bridge. He said once, 'Are you sure you want to be my partner when we come last every time? Do you want to get another partner?' And I said, 'The only time I'm going to not play with you is if you die or I die.' But every Tuesday night his wife says she can't get him to bed, because he gets all the bridge books out and he studies them, and he says, 'I can't let Flo down tomorrow.'

CL: Does he have trouble remembering how to play?

F: Completely. Bridge is a very difficult game because it has so many different conventions. And he's lost the basic rules.

CL: Does he know this about himself?

F: No, he frequently says to me, 'I can't remember anything, Flo, what's wrong with me?' And I say, 'We all can't remember things. I get up and go to the bedroom to get something and I'm standing there for two minutes thinking what did I come in here to get? That happens to everybody.'

CL: What was the happiest period of your life?

F: Probably these last few years, I've not had the stress and the problems of when you're young ... I had an easy life, really, except for the twelve years [of that first marriage]. I mean, I loved him, I thought of myself growing old with him. And that didn't pan out, so I didn't want to take another chance. I was with my second husband for five years before I married him, because he kept asking me and I kept saying no.

CL: Was [the first marriage] a very difficult break-up?

F: Yes. He had me in hospital three times, when he'd beaten me up. And I look back and I think how I hid it from so many people. And everybody loved him; he had a fantastic sense of humour. He married again, and she left him twice and refused to go back until he went to AA. [With me] he wouldn't go. I went to a place called COPE, and I met other people. They were coping with situations, and giving me advice like – if he comes home drunk, just pretend you're asleep. Well, that didn't work. Because he'd come in and pull me out of bed and throw me down the stairs. He'd say, 'Where's my dinner?' It was horrible. Horrible. It took me five years to get over it.

CL: How did you make the break in the end?

F: The last time I was in hospital I was in there for nearly four weeks, and I had a complete breakdown. I remember coming home and my mum had made this celebration lunch and invited the whole family and they were all sitting there, and I was trying to cut up my food, and my hands were shaking so much, I couldn't. And when I looked up, everybody was crying. My husband was sitting there, and he saw the situation, and I think my doctor eventually spoke to him and said, 'You need to go.' He wasn't into breaking up a marriage, but what he said to me was, 'This is what he's done to you, what are you going to do if he does this to one of the children?'

CL: Florence, it's lovely to hear you say that you're happy now at eighty-one, even with the health challenges. I think it would be uplifting for people to hear, not just that there is the possibility of a happy time later in life, but that it is possible to come through a violent marriage and find happiness again on the other side.

Ren: seventy-five
On kindness, the pleasures of being in nature and the rewards of discomfort

CL: I was thinking about the concept of the younger self, and the grief you can sometimes feel at realising you've changed. Have you experienced that? Have you wondered whether your younger self is still inside?

R: Well, you know, yes, the younger person is still there. But if I have changed at all I feel thank God I've changed, because I was so unkind when I was younger. It's not until you come into a certain age that you realise the importance of kindness. I never really had that kindness towards my mother when I was young, so I wish I'd had more of my older years to show that to her.

CL: But I wouldn't want to go back to being seventeen again.

R: Oh well, teenage is just the worst time of life.

CL: A study done in the UK about happiness has found that people report being at their happiest in their lives from fifty-nine to eighty-plus and the midlife years are the most unhappy.

R: There are happy moments in everything, but not only do you struggle with family life and all the challenges and busyness that brings, but [in midlife] you're also still in the throes of hormones.

CL: For women, that period of change is hard. Some of us get sandwiched between the teens and the ageing parents.

R: There's never any time for yourself.

CL: Once you're past those years there seem to be calmer waters.

R: There definitely is. If you ask me what is the happiest time of my life,

I've had many happy times when the kids were little, but probably it's now.

CL: Is there anything that stands out as being super important, that you would think: I have to do this really well? Or is it all like that?

R: Pretty well all like that. Family is important, of course, friendships are important, and you do your best to get it right.

CL: Health? Looking after yourself is important?

R: Yes, but I'm lucky that I enjoy it. I enjoy being physical in all different ways. I don't know what it would be like if it were a drag.

CL: I remember you talking about doing a yoga headstand, and you don't have to force yourself.

R: No, and I'm like that with a lot of stuff, like swimming. Yesterday morning I was driving back from my daughter's in Woodend, and I'd overnighted in Little Desert National Park. I wake up really early, so at the crack of dawn I had a swim in the Wimmera [River]. The moon was full and it was still up. And it's not like I have to force myself to do that, it's what I love.

CL: You were travelling in your campervan. Were you on your own?

R: I'm doing it on my own now, yes. When you ask me if I feel different to my younger self, in that respect not much has changed. Like, my body does it all right.

CL: I sometimes think this stage of life is a balancing act, keeping the past and the future in balance. Keeping stable.

R: Along with yoga, I concern myself with Buddhism. My husband was a Stoic, so that rubbed off. I think I said it to the young ones when he died: you cannot control what happens to you, you can only control how you respond to it.

CL: That's a Stoic philosophy.

R: Yes. And that is Buddhism. The other thing, be uncomfortable sometimes, because that makes you feel more alive. Don't think you have to have everything comfortable. When you're uncomfortable you actually feel more alive. It goes for physical discomfort, of course. But also for psychological discomfort. If you have to face things that hurt, are painful, it makes you think about life in different ways, you can allow yourself to be conscious of it.

CL: Sorrows have their uses?

R: Yes, although it's not always nice.

CL: That's a good thought to share. I think people would find that interesting.

R: Or annoying!

CL: It's all right for her, they'll say. But you've had your sorrows.

R: Oh yes, I've had my sorrows.

Jean: ninety
On staying active, and age as a state of mind

CL: You've seen almost a century, or coming towards a century, and a huge slice of the world. At what stage did you leave England?

J: I left in 1952, so I was going on for twenty, and I married an American.

CL: That was adventurous.

J: Yes. He was in the US Air Force. I went to America and we got married in Las Vegas. He was never in England long enough to arrange anything like a marriage. He was only there for three months at a time every couple of years.

CL: How did your family feel about you leaving?

J: They weren't very happy, but they let me go. When I look back on it now, I'd never been on a plane before, never been out of the country before. I flew on my own to New York, then Chicago, and then Los Angeles. It's a long flight, and I got airsick.

CL: Eventually, you brought your whole brood to Australia.

J: We did. Fortunately, when you retired from the American service you could go anywhere in the world and they'd ship you – furniture, car, everybody went for free. If you wanted to come back you had to pay for yourself. You could go anywhere once. Anywhere in America, or in the world, so that's what we did.

CL: I've heard about your tap dancing.

J: Yes, I did that for a good many years. I had learned when I was a kid, so I already knew how. And then I saw an ad that somebody was starting up a class – I thought I'd better go and see if I could still remember. And I did, and I was in that for a good many years. And then I met some people in there who were musicians, so we started up a little music group and I played the ukelele.

CL: You play the ukelele?

J: Yes. And we'd go out and entertain in nursing homes and retirement villages, that kind of thing. But now it's just a matter of exercising with movement, walking up and down, and marching up and down, not dancing anymore. You've really just got to keep things moving and walk when you can. I walk to the store whenever I don't have too much to carry home. It's not far to the village from here. I also do crosswords and things to keep the brain ticking over.

CL: We change over time. Do you still have a sense of that young person you were inside?

J: I think so.

CL: She's still there?

J: I think she's still in there. Maybe some people might lose that, I don't know. I say I don't feel old, well, obviously you do feel old because you can't do things that you used to do quite easily, like my driveway.

CL: That's a very steep driveway, isn't it?

J: I still can walk up the driveway, but it's harder than it used to be.

CL: Have you kept your tap shoes?

J: I've still got them, yes. I only gave it up last year. We'd given up concerts quite some time ago, but I used to do little things for the village. But the year before that I said I'm not doing it anymore. Because I don't always remember the steps quite as easily as I used to.

CL: You've always been active?

J: Yes. I can't visualise not being able to move around. I know it does happen, obviously. It helps having somebody else living with you to do small things like help open jars. It's very annoying when you're all on your own and trying to open a jar.

CL: You can put it under the hot tap.

J: I have tried that as well, and that works sometimes. Getting old is just a state of mind really. You can either allow yourself to wither away and not do anything or you can just think, well, might as well keep going while I can. Definitely try to keep moving. It's the best thing for you. Just don't settle back in the armchair and stay there.

Nicholas: seventy
On ascent rather than decline, and caring for an ageing parent

CL: You've just turned seventy. Did it feel like a big milestone?

N: Well, everyone else wanted to have parties and such, which I didn't really want at all. So I ended up having a series of small celebrations, staggered over some months, and that was quite good. But it has felt like a big thing in that I feel my life has changed. It was changing anyway. I mean, I was coming out of Covid, and coming out of retirement from the university, and with my father dying. There's change afoot, and seventy seemed to make that clear.

CL: It's a definite boundary.

N: You have different capacities. But I feel fine, and many people I know do too. I think there are a lot of positive things to be said, and even the idea of a downhill slope – of course, the end is known, but not much else is certain about when, and how. It could be an ascent of some kind.

CL: What kind of ascent do you have in mind?

N: Well, a lot of the problems of earlier life seem to have vanished, and we do have extraordinary life experience, and knowledge, and a kind of insight into things, which is very beneficial.

CL: Was there a point at which you realised you were no longer young, or began to feel old? Did that happen before seventy? Or maybe you don't feel old at all.

N: Oh, I do feel old! I think it happened earlier, maybe sixty-five, the old retirement age. But I was ready for a change, because I was working quite hard at the university and you become very aware of how old you are in that context. They start wanting to get rid of you at about fifty. You're too old; you're the wrong sort of person. You feel that coming on.

CL: And you've got a cohort of very young people that you're working with, too, and that can make you feel your age.

N: Yes, and you want to not be in the way for them.

CL: You looked after your dad in his last years.

N: Yes, pretty much. He was ninety-five when he died. He lived with his wife, not my mother. We consciously came to live near them because we knew we were into the last phase. So I was pretty closely involved.

CL: Did he remain at home?

N: He did, although he went for short stints into care, for respite, so that Mary, his wife, could go and see her kids. But it was difficult. In the end he got dehydrated, he got infections, he went into emergency and the last time he was there for two weeks, and that was it. It wasn't a harrowing end. It's been a great phase of my life, really, because I left home when I was very young, at seventeen, and didn't come back to South Australia for thirty-five years. In many ways he and I were not particularly close so just having those last years was good for both of us. We used to go out for fish and chips at Henley Beach every Thursday, and that was lovely. Among other things, that strange thing with memory and an old person where they recall things, or they talk about things that they've never talked about before. And when you're the younger one it's fascinating to get those glimpses.

Elisabeth: seventy-nine
On bereavement

CL: Can you tell me about how you've coped with the loss of your husband? I know you were very happy together, and had a wonderful family life.

E: We really understood each other, and he was always my best friend. We had a lot of respect for each other, and that's something that is in my family, so that my daughter and I respect each other greatly.

CL: The loss of that is so hard.

E: You haven't got a choice. The worst thing, when he was sick, the thing that would make me lie awake at night – I knew he was going to die, but I didn't know how and when, and that was unsettling.

CL: Were the medical people able to give you any clue?

E: We knew he had terminal cancer and there was no coming back from that. He lived a year longer than they thought he could. But, to me, I always felt I had to be strong for him. He deserved to be looked after the best we could. I had a very strong feeling of keeping it normal. I still have, and I think that's always helped me. Keep things as normal as you can, because we function better if we have some sense of normality about our lives. I needed to be strong for him, and when he died I needed to be strong for my daughter. I thought it was so sad that she'd lost her father so early, and she didn't need a mother who was in a mess. Apart from that, I thought I was lucky to still be alive. He would have done anything to live on, and here I was, still alive, so I'd better not mess it up. I'd open my curtains every day and look outside and see all the trees and the green, which I love, and think how lucky am I to still be here. You have to deal with the sadness. The sadness is there. It's hard.

CL: I don't think it ever goes, do you?

E: There are certain bits that if you think about them too much you can cry, and I think you could do that forever. But you learn to keep that down because it won't bring them back. Nothing I can do, no matter if I decided to be unhappy all my life, it wouldn't bring him back. You have to do your best for the people around you. I never wanted to pull other people down.

CL: How did you find other people dealt with it?

E: Relatively well, because *we* dealt with it well.

CL: People say that friends often avoid them afterwards because they don't know what to say.

E: There are people like that, but I understand that they don't mean any harm by it, so I didn't take offence. Generally, everyone around me was good, and I didn't want to be a wet blanket. My husband used to always ask me: 'Will you be all right when I'm gone?' And I'd always say, 'Yes, I'll be all right.' Not because I thought it would be great, but because I didn't want to worry him. Then of course, later, you think – Oh! Did I hurt his feelings?

CL: You wanted to reassure him.

E: I didn't want him worrying about me. But he had a really good attitude himself. I think we both did, and our daughter too. We had always in our family discussed the subject of death, so death was not something that, oh, that couldn't happen to us, because it can and it will at some stage. We had seen a few people close to us die, and so our daughter was well adjusted to that. It helped that I didn't have to start explaining to her why all this happened. Because it happens.

CL: There's no fairness.

E: Life is not fair, but I didn't feel the need to go there. Neither did my husband. People used to ask him sometimes, 'Do you ever say to yourself, why me?' And he'd say, 'No, this can happen to anyone, so I could say, Why not me?' He had a really good attitude. He was a beautiful man. I think the second year for me was harder. The second year is when the tears come.

CL: I've heard people say the second year is worse.

E: I think so. Because at first you're dealing with everything, and you want to be strong. The second year, people aren't around you as much because everyone has their own lives. So the second year I cried a lot. Not all day, but in little bursts. I'd have three-minute bursts of tears. That went on for some time, and then I thought, this has to stop. It has to stop. And I started taking some vitamin B for my nervous system, and after a couple of weeks it did feel better. But I had a long time, maybe five years, that when I was driving home I'd have a cry, because the memory of going home, and now he's not there anymore. I could give you a blow-by-blow account of what it was like some days, when someone's in pain and suffering. But you have to push that back, because that's not now anymore, and he's out of his suffering.

CL: It doesn't do any good to keep going over the hard parts.

E: That's what I thought when the first anniversary came up. I felt a bit nervous about that, and then I thought: the worst day was a year ago, and this day is not going to be anything like that. The worst thing has happened, so this day can never be as bad.

CL: I was going to ask how you have navigated anniversaries and birthdays.

E: The first year, I had my cousins around for a meal for his birthday. A couple of times we went out for a meal. I think you have to learn not to terrorise yourself, because this is now and that was then.

CL: That's good advice for lots of situations.

E: It's overwhelming when you first hear that something is going to kill you. You live with this right in front of your face for a while, and then you think – I can't keep doing it like this. So I used to imagine I had a cupboard behind me, and I would put those worries on a shelf in that cupboard. I knew they were there. It was right behind me, but the door was closed and I didn't have to look at it all the time. And that helped me a lot.

CL: You developed a coping strategy. I think what we're doing in managing our response to these situations, whether we're aware of it or not, is showing the younger people around us how it's possible to bear up in hard times.

E: Right from the start when he got sick, I said to my daughter, 'This is not about us, this is about him. He's the one that's got the pain. We have to try and make it as good as we can for him.' I'm an optimist by nature, and that also helped enormously. Life hands you stuff that you don't want, and you just have to suck it up. I mean, I had to learn to kill spiders. [laughter] Before, I'd yell for him: 'Spider!' He even came home from work one day because there was a big spider. But when he got sick, I thought I can't ask him to climb up there, so I'd better toughen up and learn to do it myself. So, yes, you have to toughen up. And you can make it far worse by not doing that. You

have to choose, at least I did – I can't talk for other people – you choose to be a victim or else choose to say: This has happened, give it time and it will get better. And it does. My mother had a lot of wise Dutch sayings. One of them was *naar deze tijd komt een ander*: 'after this time, comes another'.
CL: I love that.
E: And they [the ones you've lost] stay with you, anyway.

Martin: seventy-seven; Becky: seventy-three
On having Enough. On limitations, and an antifragile response to hard times

CL: I've been thinking about my resistance to travel, how it springs from a deep pleasure in home. That after a long time when you haven't felt sure where you were at home, to find a place where you do feel settled – I don't want to move from this. I know it's unadventurous.
M: In any adventure, the physical aspects of it can be tedious – but ostensibly the adventure is for the mind, and so we've just replaced those kinds of adventures with other kinds of adventures. Our minds are different now.
CL: I can have almost the same adventures through reading, and I don't have to worry about catching Covid on the plane.
B: I would say that's a kind of 'bucket list' idea of life. Do we need it? We feel, having gone to a lot of arts events, that we've had enough. We've loved going to the Venice Biennale – three times – and now we think, we don't need to go back. We've had enough. And I think that is one of the keys to our satisfaction in these years, the sense of 'Enough'.

CL: What about the limitations of age?

M: If ever I think that my lack of ability to run long distances, or lift heavy things, is a limitation, there have always been limitations – whether it's family or whether it's a job. I look at my kids and they've probably got as many [limitations] as I have, so it's not a thing just of old age. We're always constrained by something, so we've just replaced some of those constraints with others.

B: My feeling is that we've seen so many cycles of life, the good days and the bad days, the good years and the hard years – Marty and I have both lost partners to cancer; we've been through a lot of hard things – that you know that if you're having a hard time that it's going to be better. You have the peace of that experience, which some people might call wisdom. Not to get too freaked out when things are a bit rocky.

When you're in your thirties and forties and just encountering [disruption] – like a lot of these younger people during the pandemic, they lost their bundle, absolutely their mental health went to pieces. Whereas we thought, oh, this is a good chance to use the time. I wrote a book. This is like – nobody's bothering us, now what can we do? We knew that time was precious. So I think there's a kind of peace that you get at this age. Your identity is fairly formed. You are probably more of who you are, the good and the bad of that. The dross kind of goes out, and that's the beauty of the exploration of who you are in these decades towards the end. You're just being more of who you can be.

CL: What you're describing is like a refining, the refining of things and the dropping away of anything unnecessary.

B: I don't know how gold is made, but if you think about how they forge metal. We've been through some very difficult things. My first marriage was to a man who was 95 per cent paralysed, and I was with Richard for thirty-two years, so I have had a lot of challenges, and experience with disability. We made good things of that, but I think a lot of the situations, me trying to find the balance of my own creativity when someone was very dependent on me, that forges who you are. And I think that in our seventies we've been through a lot of life experiences, which make gold. But it's not handed to us on a plate.

List of Artworks

All images are original artworks by Margaret Ambridge.

'The Distance Travelled'
Charcoal on drafting film   page 10

'Homelight'
Charcoal on drafting film   page 27

'Becoming Invisible'
Indian ink and charcoal on drafting film   page 52

'Wedding Veil'
Indian ink and charcoal on drafting film   page 62

List of Artworks

'Graciously Senescing'
Indian ink and charcoal on drafting film   page 80

'Blackbird and Blossom'
Charcoal on drafting film   page 118

'Embrace'
Indian ink and charcoal on drafting film   page 136

'What is to Become of the One Who Remains?'
Charcoal on drafting film   page 149

'Gardener'
Indian ink and charcoal on drafting film   page 174

'Night Garden'
Charcoal on drafting film   page 205

'The Promise of a Second Spring'
Indian ink and charcoal on drafting film   page 222

'Blackbird'
Indian ink and charcoal on drafting film   page 236

Bibliography

Summer
Virginia Woolf. *To The Lighthouse*, London: Granada, 1977.

Chapter 1: Full Bloom
Simone de Beauvoir. *Old Age*, London: Deutsch, Weidenfeld and Nicolson, 1972.
Gransnet. 'Ageism in Fiction': http://www.gransnet.com/online-surveys-product-tests/ageism-in-fiction
Penelope Lively. *Ammonites and Leaping Fish*, London: Fig Tree, 2013.
Jean Rhys. *Wide Sargasso Sea*, England: Penguin, 1968.
—— *Good Morning, Midnight*, England: Penguin, 1969.
Susan Sontag. 'The Double Standard of Ageing', *The Other Within Us: Feminist Explorations of Women and Ageing*, ed. Marilyn Pearsall, London: Routledge, 1997.

Chapter 2: Gathering Flowers, Weaving Garlands

Colette. *Earthly Paradise*, England: Penguin, 1979.

Helen Garner. 'Dreams of Her Real Self', *Everywhere I Look*, Melbourne: Text, 2016.

Katherine Mansfield. 'Prelude', *Katherine Mansfield, The Complete Stories*, Christchurch: Golden Press, 1974.

Celia Paul. *Self Portrait*, London: Jonathan Cape, 2019.

Chapter 3: Homesick for Ourselves

Penelope Lively. *Metamorphosis*, United Kingdom: Penguin Random House, 2022.

Sarah Manguso. *Ongoingness: The End of a Diary*, United Kingdom: Picador, 2018.

Alice Munro. 'Bardon Bus', *The Moons of Jupiter*, England: Penguin Books, 1983.

—— 'Labor Day Dinner', *The Moons of Jupiter*, England: Penguin Books, 1983.

Cheryl Strayed. 'What You Know Changes': https://cherylstrayed.substack.com/p/what-you-know-changes

Chapter 4: Disappearing Acts

Akiko Busch. *How to Disappear*, New York: Penguin Press, 2019.

Germaine Greer. 'Serenity and Power', *The Other Within Us: Feminist Explorations of Women and Ageing,* ed. Marilyn Pearsall, London: Routledge, 1997.

John Ruskin. *Selected Writings*, Oxford: Oxford University Press, 2004.

Vita Sackville-West. *All Passion Spent*, London: Virago Press, 1983.

Sally Vickers. *Miss Garnet's Angel*, London and New York: Fourth Estate, 2000.

Deborah Wood. 'Society "Disappears" Ageing Women': http://www.unwomenmag.com/society-disappears-ageing-women-so-i-harnessed-that-cloak-of-invisibility-to-do-all-sorts-of-inappropriate-things-deborah-wood/

Autumn

Virginia Woolf. *To the Lighthouse*, London: Granada, 1977.

Chapter 5: Death Cleaning

Margareta Magnusson. *The Gentle Art of Swedish Death Cleaning*, London: Scribe, 2017.

Chapter 7: Past and Future in Every Moment

Jorge Luis Borges. *Labyrinths: Selected Stories and Other Writings*, New York: New Directions, 1964.

Marian Halligan. 'Cherubs', *The Worry Box*, Melbourne: Minerva, 1993.

Nathaniel Hawthorne. 'The Haunted Mind', *Twice Told Tales*, Philadelphia, David McKay, 1889: https://www.gutenberg.org/cache/epub/13707/pg13707-images.html

Tamara Kohn. 'Waiting on Death Row', *Waiting*, Melbourne: Melbourne University Press, 2009.

Doris Lessing. *Diary of a Good Neighbour*, London: Michael Joseph, 1984.

Rosemary Robins. 'Waiting for Rain in the Goulburn Valley', *Waiting*, Melbourne: Melbourne University Press, 2009.

Vita Sackville-West. *All Passion Spent*, London: Virago Press, 1983.

Susan Sontag. 'A Letter to Borges', *Where the Stress Falls*, London: Jonathan Cape, 2002.

Michael Steinman, ed. *The Element of Lavishness: Letters of Sylvia Townsend Warner and William Maxwell*, New York: Counterpoint, 2001.

Gillian G Tan. 'Senses of Waiting Among Tibetan Nomads', *Waiting*, Melbourne: Melbourne University Press, 2009.

Virginia Woolf. *Mrs Dalloway*, London: Vintage, 2000.

Chapter 8: The Possibility of Radiance

Liz Byrski. *Getting On: Some Thoughts on Women and Ageing*, Sydney: Momentum, 2012.

Betty Friedan. *The Fountain of Age*, London: Jonathan Cape, 1993.

Doris Lessing. *The Diaries of Jane Somers*, London: Michael Joseph, 1984.

May Sarton. *At Seventy: A Journal*, New York: Open Road Media, 2014.

—— *At Eighty-Two: A Journal*, New York: Open Road Media, 2014.

Patti Smith. *M Train*, London: Bloomsbury, 2015.

Susan Sontag. 'The Double Standard of Ageing', *The Other Within Us: Feminist Explorations of Women and Ageing*, ed. Marilyn Pearsall, London: Routledge, 1997.

Michael Steinman, ed. *The Element of Lavishness: Letters of Sylvia Townsend Warner and William Maxwell*, New York: Counterpoint, 2001.

Charlotte Wood. *The Weekend*, Sydney: Allen and Unwin, 2019.

Winter
Virginia Woolf. *Night and Day*, Oxford: Blackwell, 1994.

Chapter 9: When Enough Is Enough
Ernest Becker. *The Denial of Death*, New York: Free Press, c. 1973.
Georgia Blain. *The Museum of Words: A Memoir of Language, Writing and Mortality*, Melbourne: Scribe, 2017.
Ronald Blythe. *The View in Winter: Reflections on Old Age*, Hammondsworth: Penguin, 1981.
JM Coetzee. 'When a Woman Grows Old', *The Pole*, Melbourne: Text, 2023.
Katherine Tamiko Arguile. 'The Rich World Within: Vale Alison Flett': https://inreview.com.au/inreview/2023/09/22/the-rich-world-within-vale-alison-flett/
'Terror Management Theory', *Psychology Today*: http://www.psychologytoday.com/intl/basics/terror-management-theory

Chapter 10: Saying Goodbye
Beryl Markham. *West With the Night*, London: Virago, 1984.

Chapter 11: Lost in Time
Patricia Bauer and Marina Larkina. 'Childhood Amnesia in the Making', *Journal of Experimental Psychology*: https://doi.org/10.1037/a0033307
Nora Ephron. *I Remember Nothing*, New York: Alfred A Knopf, 2010.
Melanie Joosten. *A Long Time Coming: Essays on Old Age*, Melbourne: Scribe, 2016.

Fiona McFarlane. *The Night Guest*, Melbourne: Penguin, 2013.
Mary Pipher. *Women Rowing North*, New York: Bloomsbury, 2019.
May Sarton. *At Seventy: A Journal*, New York: Open Road Media, 2014.

Chapter 12: Love and Age

Leonora Carrington. *The Hearing Trumpet*, Great Britain: Routledge & Kegan Paul, 1977.
Kent Haruf. *Our Souls at Night*, Sydney: Pan Macmillan, 2016.
Alice Munro. 'The Bear Came Over the Mountain', *Family Furnishings*, New York: Alfred A Knopf, 2014.
Elizabeth Strout. *Olive Kitteridge*, Great Britain: Simon and Schuster, 2011.
—— *Anything Is Possible*, United Kingdom: Penguin Random House, 2018.

Chapter 13: The View from the Tower

Frieda Fromm-Reichmann. 'Loneliness', *Contemporary Psychoanalysis*, 1990: https://psptraining.com/wp-content/uploads/Fromm-ReichmannF.-CPS_Loneliness.pdf
Olivia Laing. *The Lonely City*, Great Britain: Canongate, 2017.
Carol Lefevre. *The Tower*, Australia: Spinifex, 2022.
Haruki Murakami. 'A Walk to Kobe': https://granta.com/a-walk-to-kobe
Rainer Maria Rilke. 'Go to the Limits of Your Longing', *The Book of Hours*, translated and with an introduction and notes by Annemarie S Kidder, Evanston: Northwestern University Press, 2001.
Nassim Nicholas Taleb. *Antifragile: Things that Gain from Disorder*, United States: Random House, 2012.

Chapter 14: Finding Shelter

Ashleigh Barraclough. 'Communal Living Is Growing in Australia. Residents Say It Can Create Community and Reduce Cost of Living': https://www.abc.net.au/news/2022-07-22/communal-living-reduce-cost-of-living-loneliness/101146464

Karen L Fingerman. 'Millennials and Their Parents: Implications of the New Young Adulthood for Midlife Adults', *Innovation in Aging*, Volume 1, Issue 3, November 2017: https://academic.oup.com//innovateage/article/1/3/igx026/4643095

Tom Wolfe. 'The 'Me' Decade and the Third Great Awakening', *New York Magazine*: https://nymag.com/article/tom-wolfe-me-decade-third-great-awakening.html

Spring

Virginia Woolf. *A Room of One's Own*, Great Britain: Grafton Books, 1977.

Chapter 15: Imagined Gardens

Sylvia Ashton-Warner. *Spinster*, London: Virago, 1980.

Colette. *Earthly Paradise*, England: Penguin, 1979.

Nicholas Culpeper. *Culpeper's Complete Herbal & English Physician*, London: Parkgate Books, 1997.

Penelope Hobhouse. *Gertrude Jekyll on Gardening: An Anthology*, London: Macmillan, 1985.

Vita Sackville-West and Sarah Raven. *Vita Sackville-West's Sissinghurst*. London: Virago, 2014.

Chapter 16: Russian Dolls and Roses
Carol Lefevre. *The Happiness Glass*, Australia: Spinifex Press, 2018.
Doris Lessing. *Diary of a Good Neighbour*, London: Michael Joseph, 1984.
Kate Llewellyn. *A Fig at the Gate*, Sydney: Allen and Unwin, 2014.
Charlotte Wood. *The Weekend*, Sydney: Allen and Unwin, 2019.

Chapter 18: The Homeward Star
Joan Didion. 'On Keeping a Notebook', *Slouching Towards Bethlehem*, London: Flamingo, 2001.
John Ruskin. *John Ruskin, Selected Writings*, ed. Dinah Birch, Oxford: Oxford University Press, 2004.
Michael Steinman, ed. *The Element of Lavishness: Letters of Sylvia Townsend Warner and William Maxwell*, New York: Counterpoint, 2001.
Sue Stuart-Smith. *The Well Gardened Mind*, London: William Collins, 2020.

Chapter 20: Okay, Bloomer
Henri Bergson. *Time and Free Will*, trans. FL Pogson, London: Swan, Sonnenschein, 1910.
Thich Nhat Hanh. *No Mud, No Lotus*, California: Parallax Press, 2014.
Elizabeth Lawrence. *Through the Garden Gate*, United States: University of North Carolina Press, 1995.
Mary Pipher. *Women Rowing North*, New York: Bloomsbury, 2019.
Helen Small. *The Long Life*, Oxford: Oxford University Press, 2007.

Acknowledgements

Earlier versions of four of the chapters in *Bloomer* were commissioned as essays for *The Conversation* and re-published on various news outlets. 'Love and Age', under the title 'Love in the Time of Incontinence: Why young people don't have a monopoly on love, or even sex', was re-published by Thames and Hudson in *A Year of Consequence*, edited by Justin Bergman. I am indebted to Jo Case for her patience and the sharp editorial eye she brought to those early essays, and I am especially grateful for her unstinting encouragement to collect the pieces into a longer work. An extract from 'The Homeward Star' appeared in the anthology *Not Dead Yet* (Spinifex Press), and an extract from my prose chapbook *Of Bread and Roses* forms part of 'The Ordinary and Extraordinary'.

During the writing I talked to many older people about their experiences of ageing. The stories they shared with me – a complete

Acknowledgements

stranger in most cases – inspired me to persevere whenever the project threatened to implode. Their courage and optimism informed the writing, and I am indebted to each and every one of them for their generosity. In the end those conversations generated almost enough material for another book, which meant that only extracts could be included here. I hope to make the conversations accessible in full on my website, but my further hope is that the things we discussed over cups of tea might help spark a wider discussion about ageing and ageism.

Recording and transcribing those chats was supported by a grant from Arts South Australia, which also funded the development of the artworks by Margaret Ambridge. The validation of the project this funding implied was much appreciated at a time when the work that lay ahead felt overwhelming.

Lauren Cortis patiently demystified the voluntary assisted dying process for me. Darlene O'Leary was equally patient in teasing out the elements at work in the lives of older women forced into homelessness, especially those who cross the threshold at Adelaide's Catherine House. Hayley Everuss at The Loneliness Project shed light on the adverse effects of loneliness on people of all kinds in our communities, and the ways in which we might try to remedy their suffering.

I'd like to thank Adrian Howard for his permission to quote the poem 'Unbearable Lightness' by his late partner, the gifted poet Alison Flett.

Writing can be lonely at times, and I have appreciated Margaret Ambridge's companionship. As well as responding to my writing with her exquisite artworks, she put me in touch with people who contributed their thoughts on ageing. It was through one of Margaret's neighbours that I was welcomed into Bronte's garden and spent time there at twilight with Bronte's gardener, who shared his knowledge of the layers of time at work in a garden landscape. Margaret's partner Mark generously offered his technical expertise to digitise the artworks.

A book that you can hold in your hands is always an outcome of the special energies and skills of many people. My gratitude is due to all at Affirm Press who have helped shepherd *Bloomer* into the world, and especially to Martin Hughes. I feel fortunate that our paths crossed when they did, and my heartfelt thanks goes to Pip Williams for the introduction. Martin's enthusiasm and vision for this book and his perceptive reading of it at the structural stage have been crucial to the way it has come together. Emma Schwarcz's subtle and exacting editing has been another vital factor: Emma helped untangle my thinking in many places, and her work has made *Bloomer* the best it could be. Kevin O'Brien was ever-patient as he expertly guided this project towards print. If all that weren't enough, the gorgeous cover design by George Saad sparks joy in my heart every time I look at it.

To my agent, Fran Moore, always intrepid in the trenches, thank you for guiding this manuscript over all the rocky patches until it found the perfect home.

Finally, to my two dear ones, Christopher and Rafael Lefevre, thank you for everything. Your presence in my life is my greatest blessing.